Correction of Severe Foot and Ankle Deformities

Editor

ANDY MOLLOY

FOOT AND ANKLE CLINICS

www.foot.theclinics.com

Consulting Editor
MARK S. MYERSON

June 2020 • Volume 25 • Number 2

ELSEVIER

1600 John F. Kennedy Boulevard • Suite 1800 • Philadelphia, Pennsylvania, 19103-2899

http://www.theclinics.com

FOOT AND ANKLE CLINICS Volume 25, Number 2
June 2020 ISSN 1083-7515, ISBN-978-0-323-71295-8

Editor: Lauren Boyle
Developmental Editor: Nicole Congleton

Foot and Ankle Clinics (ISSN 1083-7515) is published quarterly by Elsevier, Inc., 360 Park Avenue South, New York, NY 10010-1710. Months of issue are March, June, September, and December. Periodicals postage paid at New York, NY, and additional mailing offices. Subscription price per year is $340.00 (US individuals), $582.00 (US institutions), $100.00 (US students), $371.00 (Canadian individuals), $669.00 (Canadian institutions), $100.00 (Canadian students), $470.00 (international individuals), $669.00 (international institutions), and $215.00 (international students). To receive student/resident rate, orders must be accompanied by name of affiliated institution, date of term, and the *signature* of program/residency coordinator on institution letterhead. Orders will be billed at individual rate until proof of status is received. Foreign air speed delivery is included in all *Clinics* subscription prices. All prices are subject to change without notice. **POSTMASTER:** Send address changes to *Foot and Ankle Clinics*, Elsevier Health Sciences Division, Subscription Customer Service, 3251 Riverport Lane, Maryland Heights, MO 63043. **Customer Service: 1-800-654-2452 (US and Canada). From outside of the United States and Canada, call 314-447-8871. Fax: 314-447-8029. E-mail: JournalsCustomerService-usa@ elsevier.com (for print support); JournalsOnlineSupport-usa@elsevier.com (for online support).**

Reprints. For copies of 100 or more, of articles in this publication, please contact the Commercial Reprints Department, Elsevier Inc., 360 Park Avenue South, New York, NY 10010-1710. Tel.: 212-633-3874; Fax: 212-633-3820; E-mail: reprints@elsevier.com.

Contributors

CONSULTING EDITOR

MARK S. MYERSON, MD
Executive Director and Founder, Steps2Walk, Baltimore, Maryland, USA

EDITOR

ANDY MOLLOY, MBChB, MRCS, FRCS Tr&Orth
Consultant Orthopaedic Surgeon, Trauma and Orthopaedics, Aintree University Hospital, Honorary Clinical Senior Lecturer, Department of Musculoskeletal Biology, University of Liverpool, Consultant Orthopaedic Surgeon, Spire Liverpool, Liverpool, United Kingdom

AUTHORS

SAMUEL B. ADAMS, MD
Associate Residency Program Director, Co-Chief, Division of Foot and Ankle Surgery, Director of Foot and Ankle Research, Assistant Professor, Department of Orthopaedic Surgery, Duke University Medical Center, Durham, North Carolina, USA

ALON BURG, MD
Department of Orthopedic Surgery, Foot and Ankle Service, Rabin Medical Center, Petah Tikva, Sackler Faculty of Medicine, Tel Aviv University, Tel Aviv, Israel

MARK B. DAVIES, BM, FRCS, FRCS (Tr & Orth)
Consultant in Foot and Ankle Surgery, Foot and Ankle Unit, Northern General Hospital, Foot and Ankle Consultants' Office, Sheffield, United Kingdom

ASHTIN DOORGAKANT, MBBS, FRCS (Tr & Orth)
Senior Foot and Ankle Fellow, Foot and Ankle Unit, Northern General Hospital, Foot and Ankle Offices, Sheffield, United Kingdom

NORMAN ESPINOSA, MD
Institute for Foot and Ankle Reconstruction, Fussinstitut Zurich, Zurich, Switzerland

BEN FISCHER, BSc (Hons), MBChB (Hons), FRCS (Tr&Orth)
Trauma and Orthopaedic Consultant, Trauma and Orthopaedic Department, Aintree University Hospital, Liverpool, United Kingdom; Mersey Ortho-Plastic Group, Liverpool Limb Reconstruction Service

GAVIN HEYES, FRCS, MSc
Consultant, Department of Trauma and Orthopaedic Surgery, Aintree University Hospital, Liverpool, United Kingdom

SHUYUAN LI, MD, PhD
Program Coordinator, Steps2Walk, Baltimore, Maryland, USA

CHRISTINE MARX, MD
University Hospital Carl Gustav Carus, TU Dresden, Dresden, Germany

LYNDON WILLIAM MASON, MB BCh, MRCS (eng), FRCS (Tr&Orth), FRCS (Glasg)
Foot and Ankle Trauma Lead, Trauma and Orthopaedic Department, Aintree University Hospital, Musculoskeletal System Lead, Honorary Senior Clinical Lecturer, University of Liverpool, Liverpool, United Kingdom

ANDY MOLLOY, MBChB, MRCS, FRCS Tr&Orth
Consultant Orthopaedic Surgeon, Trauma and Orthopaedics, Aintree University Hospital, Honorary Clinical Senior Lecturer, Department of Musculoskeletal Biology, University of Liverpool, Consultant Orthopaedic Surgeon, Spire Liverpool, Liverpool, United Kingdom

C. LUCAS MYERSON, MD
Department of Orthopaedic Surgery, Penn Medicine, Philadelphia, Pennsylvania, USA

MARK S. MYERSON, MD
Executive Director and Founder, Steps2Walk, Baltimore, Maryland, USA

EZEQUIEL PALMANOVICH, MD
Orthopedic Department, Director of the Foot and Ankle Service, Meir Medical Service, Kfar Saba, Sackler Faculty of Medicine, Tel Aviv University, Tel Aviv, Israel

NICHOLAS PETERSON, MBChB (Hons), FRCS (Orth)
Royal Liverpool and Broadgreen University Hospital, Alder Hey Children's Hospital, Liverpool, United Kingdom

MICHAEL S. PINZUR, MD
Professor of Orthopedic Surgery and Rehabilitation, Loyola University Health System, Maywood, Illinois, USA

CHRISTOPHER PRIOR, MBChB, FRCS (Orth)
Alder Hey Children's Hospital, Liverpool, United Kingdom

STEFAN RAMMELT, MD, PhD
Professor, Head of the Foot and Ankle Center, University Hospital Carl Gustav Carus, TU Dresden, Dresden, Germany

STEPHAN H. WIRTH, MD
Department of Orthopaedics, University of Zurich, The Balgrist, Zurich, Switzerland

Editorial Advisory Board

Contents

The severe foot and ankle deformities the authors' organization has encountered in humanitarian programs worldwide are more complicated than those surgeons treat in daily practice in developed countries. Severity of deformity, patients' economic limitations, patients' expectations and realistic needs in life, availability of surgical instrumentation, the local team's understanding of foot and ankle surgery and their ability to do consultation for patients postoperatively, and compliance of patients all account for success of the surgery. Regardless of the effort surgeons make, complications and recurrence occur. Educating and training local surgeons to take over medical care are the most important goals of the programs.

Clubfoot is a complex 4-dimensional deformity involving the hindfoot, midfoot, and forefoot. The fourth dimension is time. Treatment aims at achieving a pain-free, plantigrade, and mobile foot but, over time, flexible deformities become fixed and more difficult to manage. The Ponseti method of serial manipulation and casting can be used successfully in older children and may reduce the need for extensive open surgery. Alternatively, gradual correction of by an external device enables simultaneous correction of all components of the deformity without shortening the foot. Combining gradual soft tissue distraction with open releases and/or bony procedures may achieve a pain-free and plantigrade foot.

Malunion of ankle and pilon fractures has significant detrimental effect on function and development of post-trauma osteoarthritis. Unfortunately, the incidence of malunion has been reported to be increasing. It is important to assess the ankle for congruency, because this determines the level where correction will occur. A plethora of techniques are available, with low-level evidence supporting each, and therefore it is important that the treating surgeon is fully prepared and comfortable in the techniques they are to use. Supplementary procedures are common and should be expected. This article provides a review of current methods of treatment and their outcomes.

Severe calcaneal malunions are debilitating conditions owing to substantial hindfoot deformity with subtalar arthritis and soft tissue imbalance. Type III malunions are best treated with a subtalar distraction bone block fusion. Additional osteotomies may be required for severe varus or superior displacement of the calcaneal tuberosity. Type IV malunions result from malunited calcaneal fracture-dislocations and require a 3-dimensional corrective osteotomy. Type V malunions warrant additional ankle debridement and reconstruction of the calcaneal shape to provide support for the talus in the ankle mortise. Accompanying soft tissue procedures include Achilles tendon lengthening, peroneal tendon release, and rerouting behind the lateral malleolus.

This article provides an overview regarding the virtual planning and precise execution of corrective osteotomies around the foot and ankle. Based on 3-dimensional data obtained from CT scans, surgeons are able to create a virtual plan of how to correct a complex deformity. This plan is transferred into the production of true patient-specific guides, designed to perform a specific surgical intervention. The authors have extensive experience with this technique and were involved in the development of the method. The current article provides an overview regarding the virtual planning and precise execution of corrective osteotomies around the foot and ankle.

Stage 4 flatfoot represents only a small proportion of flatfoot cases and is likely to become even rarer. The evidence base to guide treatment is limited to case series and expert opinion. Therefore, a pragmatic approach to treatment must be taken. Low-demand individuals may manage well with conservative treatment. Surgical management is complex, likely to require staging, and has a significant complication profile. Patients should be fully informed and understanding of this. First principles of surgery should be followed, including restoring hindfoot and ankle joint alignment, appropriate soft tissue balancing, and optimizing function by limiting arthrodeses and subsequent stiffness.

Salvage arthrodesis for failed total ankle replacement can be a successful procedure. The decision to perform salvage arthrodesis is based on many factors, but the following are the most important indications: severe loss of bonestock (tibia, talus, or both), inadequate soft tissue coverage, or the inability to eradicate an infection. With few revision implants on the market, salvage arthrodesis is currently the most common treatment for failed replacement and justification for revision ankle replacement is limited when any of these factors are present.

Treatment of Ankle and Hindfoot Charcot Arthropathy

Michael S. Pinzur

It is now well accepted that diabetic patients with clinically and radio-graphically nonplantigrade Charcot foot arthropathy are best managed with correction of the acquired deformity. Several investigations have demonstrated a high probability for a favorable clinical outcome when the deformity is in the midfoot. Unstable deformity at the subtalar or ankle joints portends a far worse clinical outcome. The goal of this discussion was to describe the author's approach to this highly challenging clinical problem.

Managing the Complex Cavus Foot Deformity

Mark S. Myerson and C. Lucas Myerson

This article describes approaches to and the management of complex cavus foot deformities. Correction of rigid multiplanar deformities can be very challenging, given the presence of skeletal deformities in multiple planes and combined with a varying degree of muscle imbalance. The complexity of these cases always requires a case-by-case approach. Some of the cases presented here occur in patients who have previously undergone surgical management for their deformity, several of which are complicated by additional deformities. With a firm understanding and application of the principles of deformity correction, however, one may reliably offer satisfactory results.

An Approach to Managing Midfoot Charcot Deformities

Ashtin Doorgakant and Mark B. Davies

We present an approach to managing complex deformities in Charcot neuroarthropathy that typically present around the midfoot. This approach follows a stepwise progression from prevention, early detection, nonoperative through to operative management. It centers on multidisciplinary care with input from diabetologists, orthotists, plaster technicians, physiotherapists, orthopedic, vascular, and/or plastic surgeons. We discuss the timing of surgery with regard to Eichenholtz stage of disease and trends toward early surgical intervention. We review traditional and new surgical concepts. We evaluate the role of limited interventions. We aim to provide a template for deciding where future research priorities should be directed.

Correction of Severe Hallux Valgus with Metatarsal Adductus Applying the Concepts of Minimally Invasive Surgery

Alon Burg and Ezequiel Palmanovich

The combination of hallux valgus and metatarsus adductus presents a surgical challenge even for the experienced foot and ankle surgeon, as the position of the lesser metatarsals restricts the space for metatarsal head displacement. We describe the application of concepts of minimally invasive techniques to correct this deformity. Proximal metatarsal osteotomy to correct the position of lesser metatarsals, followed by minimally invasive bunion surgery, shows promising results. In a short series, proximal metatarsal osteotomy showed excellent correction of the deformity. At final follow-up, all the deformed feet consolidated in correct positions.

FOOT AND ANKLE CLINICS

RELATED SERIES

Clinics in Sports Medicine
Orthopedic Clinics
Physical Medicine and Rehabilitation Clinics

THE CLINICS ARE NOW AVAILABLE ONLINE!
Access your subscription at:
www.theclinics.com

Erratum

https://www.foot.theclinics.com/article/S1083-7515(19)30095-6/fulltext; https://www.foot.theclinics.com/article/S1083-7515(19)30135-4/fulltext; https://www.foot.theclinics.com/article/S1083-7515(19)30115-9/fulltext.

In the December 2019 issue, in the article "State of the Art in Lesser Metatarsophalangeal Instability," (pages 627-640) and in the March 2020 issue, in the articles "Controversies in the Approach to Complex Hallux Valgus Correction," (pages xv-xvi), "Management of Hallux Valgus in Metatarsus Adductus," (pages 59-68) the author's affiliation was incorrect. It should be Sudheer Reddy, MD, Shady Grove Orthopaedics, Department of Orthopaedic Surgery, Adventist Medical Center, 9601 Blackwell Road, Suite 100, Rockville, MD 20850, USA.

Foot Ankle Clin N Am 25 (2020) xiii
https://doi.org/10.1016/j.fcl.2020.04.003

Preface

Correction of Severe Foot and Ankle Deformities

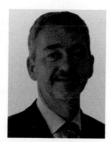

Andy Molloy, MBChB, MRCS, FRCS Tr&Orth
Editor

For the majority of Orthopedic Foot and Ankle surgeons, there is a wide range in the complexity and nature of cases due to the huge variance of conditions we treat.

Severe deformity correction of the foot, ankle, or both is a hugely rewarding surgical challenge. However, it can also be a daunting task, especially in multiplanar deformities or in the presence of defects or neurologic abnormalities. Because of the wide extent of deformities as well as of their causality, it can be difficult for a single surgeon to have consistent expertise in surgical treatment of such deformities.

All of the authors in this issue of *Foot and Ankle Clinics of North America* are experts in dealing with their respective topics. I strongly commend them for their time, effort, and articles on such wide-ranging issues as neurologic conditions, and posttraumatic and postsurgical deformities. They have succeeded in their remit to provide an algorithmic approach in dealing with these most severe of conditions so as to help surgeons, and their patients, in the decision-making process in developing a successful surgical strategy. These include wide-ranging techniques from minimally invasive to fusion surgery, from internal to complex external fixation as well as from 3D printed guides and prostheses to operating in humanitarian programs with little available fixation techniques.

It is an honor to be guest editor for this issue of *Foot and Ankle Clinics of North America* on Correction of Severe Foot and Ankle Deformities. As always, a huge thanks go to the staff from Elsevier in their help in putting the issue together as well to Dr Myerson for his huge support, assistance, and expertise.

Foot Ankle Clin N Am 25 (2020) xv–xvi
https://doi.org/10.1016/j.fcl.2020.04.001
1083-7515/20/© 2020 Published by Elsevier Inc.

I sincerely hope that you enjoy this issue of this issue of *Foot and Ankle Clinics of North America* and that it is of significant benefit to you and your patients.

Andy Molloy, MBChB, MRCS, FRCS Tr&Orth
Trauma and Orthopaedics
University Hospital Aintree
Liverpool L9 7AL

Department of Musculoskeletal Biology
University of Liverpool

Spire Liverpool
57 Greenbank Road
Liverpool, L18 1HQ, UK

E-mail address:
andymolloy3@gmail.com

Managing Severe Foot and Ankle Deformities in Global Humanitarian Programs

Shuyuan Li, MD, PhD, Mark S. Myerson, MD*

KEYWORDS

- Foot and ankle • Deformity • Humanitarian program • Steps2Walk • Clubfoot
- Calcaneovalgus • Ball-and-socket ankle • Cavovarus

KEY POINTS

- This article presents a variety of severe deformities that the authors have encountered on Steps2Walk humanitarian programs globally.
- In correcting foot and ankle deformities, treatment should include both bony alignment correction and soft tissue balance.
- On a humanitarian medical care mission, foot and ankle surgeons have to take into consideration the severity of the deformity, the patients' economic limitations, patients' expectations and realistic needs in life, availability of surgical instrumentation, the local team's understanding of foot and ankle surgery and their ability to do continuous consultation for patients postoperatively, compliance of the patients, and how they will cope if bilateral surgery is performed.
- Limited essential continuous follow-up always is one of the top problems that can cause complications and recurrence in an area where there is not adequate orthopedic foot and ankle surgery follow-up. Therefore, educating and training local surgeons to take over the future medical care are the most important goals of the authors' global humanitarian programs.

INTRODUCTION

This article presents a variety of severe deformities that the authors have encountered in Steps2Walk humanitarian programs globally. Many of these deformities are not seen routinely in the Western world today and provide unique challenges for treatment and correction.[1] There are differences in the expectations of the patients whom the authors treat compared with those in the Western world; the latter have different goals, some of which may be quite unrealistic in these programs. Many of the deformities discussed have been present since birth, whereas others are caused by systemic disease, neuromuscular disorders, trauma, and so forth. In many parts of the world,

Steps2Walk, 1209 Harbor Island Walk, Baltimore, MD 21230, USA
* Corresponding author.
E-mail address: Mark4feet@aol.com

Foot Ankle Clin N Am 25 (2020) 183–203
https://doi.org/10.1016/j.fcl.2020.01.001
1083-7515/20/© 2020 Elsevier Inc. All rights reserved.

foot.theclinics.com

there is an acceptance of these deformities due to patients' financial problems or the limited availability of orthopedic foot and ankle surgery in the local areas. Most patients have learned to live with a deformity and accept the disability, until the authors have been able to provide treatment through humanitarian projects. In treating these patients, in addition to careful systematic clinical assessment, a thorough communication with the patient and the family, with a good understanding of the local culture and the patient's background, can never be overemphasized. For a majority of these patients, a plantigrade foot always is desirable,[2] but for some, the ability to wear a shoe is more important than obtaining a perfectly shaped and aligned foot, which may be not only unnecessary but also unrealistic given the equipment that the authors are working with. Having said this, the authors always attempt to obtain the best possible correction so that the patient is able to ambulate and wear a shoe.

As always, treatment should include both bony alignment correction and soft tissue balance whenever necessary. For flexible pediatric, in particular congenital, deformities, osteotomies are preferable, even for severe deformities. Arthrodesis usually is reserved for severe rigid deformities in adults. There often are exceptions, however, where the authors are forced to perform a hindfoot arthrodesis or talectomy in a child with severe rigid deformity. The authors have to take into consideration the recovery, the ability of the patient to obtain rehabilitation, their ability to return for follow-up visits, and how they will cope if bilateral surgery is performed. For many of these patients, bilateral surgery is preferable, but many of them live in rural areas where ambulation even with crutches is difficult on uneven terrain, and it is difficult to obtain a wheelchair for them. Family resources must be taken into consideration when planning these surgeries.

During the surgeries, the authors often are confronted with a lack of resources, mostly with respect to implants and power equipment, which are taken for granted in day-to-day practice in the Western world. The authors frequently use solely Kirschner wires of various diameters to maintain stability after deformity correction. In some countries, the authors have been fortunate to have corporate support for the use of plates and screws, which make the recovery a little easier. The authors have found, however, that wires work extraordinarily well both for children and in adults.[3,4] Although external fixation with staged correction may be ideal for severe deformities to avoid potential wound and neurovascular complications, which are higher in 1-stage correction,[5–7] it is not preferred in patients from rural areas, where postoperative medical care is limited. In such cases, 1-stage careful aggressive correction is ideal to obtain definite outcome and avoid complications as much as possible. Sometimes, surgeons need to accept that a functional foot with some minor residual deformities is more realistic than perfect alignment with procedures that carry a higher risk of complications.,

UNTREATED CLUBFOOT

Clubfoot deformity refers to a variety and range of deformities that cause continuing disability of the hindfoot and ankle and, in the most severe cases, patients are load bearing on 1 side of the foot and ankle. There are several subcategories of deformity, including equinus, calcaneus, varus, valgus, adductus, and abductus. The etiology of these varied deformities can be congenital, caused by multiple vascular deficiencies, position in utero, abnormal congenital muscle insertion, and genetic factors, or be associated with neuromuscular disorders, such as poliomyelitis, cerebral palsy, arthrogryposis, and spinal bifida.[8–11] Neglected or untreated clubfoot deformities are common in developing countries and regions where there are limited pediatric orthopedic resources and a high rate of recurrent deformity due to recidivism and inability to return for follow-up treatments. van Wijicke and colleagues[12] did a qualitative and partly quantitative study with semistructured interviews in 4 countries—the Netherlands, South Africa, Argentina, and Indonesia—with both caregivers, mostly parents of children with clubfoot, and practitioners treating clubfoot. They found that poverty, long travel duration, and beliefs of supernatural were the most common causes for the delay of treatment of clubfeet. It was proposed by the investigators that accessible clinics in rural areas could be good alternatives to highly specialized hospitals in large cities.[12] This is exactly the goal of the global humanitarian educational projects of Steps2Walk. The authors are coordinating global orthopedic foot and ankle surgery resources to deliver professional education to local orthopedic surgeons and medical care to patients.

In neglected clubfoot cases, usually there is severe stiffness caused by long-standing soft tissue contracture or even arthritis. Therefore, surgeries usually are indicated, including soft tissue release, Achilles tendon lengthening, tenotomies, tendon transfer, triple arthrodesis, and talectomy with or without tibiocalcaneal arthrodesis.[13–15] Soft tissue procedures alone usually do not provide adequate correction; therefore, bony procedures usually are needed to sustain the correction.[15] Ghali and colleagues[16] reviewed 125 patients with 194 feet affected by congenital talipes equinovarus deformity treated during the period 1959 to 1980. In the early group of 70 patients, who presented within 4 weeks of birth, the investigators reported excellent or good results in 94% of feet treated conservatively and 82% of feet that required pantalar release. In the late group of 55 patients who presented after 4 weeks of birth, satisfactory results were achieved in 75% of cases. The investigators found there was no statistical correlation between early soft tissue release and a good final outcome, but there was a positive statistical correlation between good clinical results and a high talocalcaneal index. The external fixation technique has the ability to correct all deformity components of rigid deformity at the same time without bone resection or limb shortening. Complications, however, such as pin tract infection, early consolidation, and articular subluxation, all are concerns, in particular among patients from areas without adequate medical care and where sequential postoperative follow-up is unavailable.[13,17,18] Among bony procedures, triple arthrodesis is an option for skeletally mature patients with rigid clubfoot deformity. There is a high incidence of complications, however, with long-term follow-up, including residual deformities, degenerative osteoarthritis, and nonunion.[19,20] There also are opinions claiming that triple arthrodesis is not the first choice for patients with a neurologic foot deformity, because of the dangers of joint degeneration and skin ulceration caused by the stiffness of the foot.[21]

Talectomy has been used to treat clubfoot since the seventeenth century.[22] More recently it has been widely used when reduction of the deformity is extremely difficult or when the talus is very deformed.[23] It is stated that talectomy could provide sufficient laxity for the hindfoot deformity to be corrected without tension. The tibiocalcaneal pseudoarthrosis that is created remains stable and relatively congruous with a plantigrade foot with little tendency to relapse due to the stable position and the absence of medial tension.[14] According to El-Sherbini and Omran,[15] in a 10-year prospective observational study, talectomy is a relatively straightforward technique, which allows early mobilization of the operated extremity, and an effective procedure for correction of severe rigid equinovarus feet with significant effect, provided the talus is completely removed and the calcaneus can be aligned in the ankle mortise. Cooper and colleagues followed a series of 26 talectomy cases who had the surgery at an average age of 10.25 years for an average of 20 years. The results were good with obtaining stable and painless plantigrade feet, regardless of the preoperative deformities. They believed that talectomy is indicated only in rigid and severe deformed feet, whereas other less radical approaches are not recommended for various reasons.[24]

The authors present a 28-year old woman with untreated bilateral club foot deformities. There was no movement of either foot whatsoever, and the ankle also was extremely rigid. The options for treatment included a talectomy combined with a tibiocalcaneal arthrodesis, a talectomy without an arthrodesis, or correction of the feet gradually with an external fixator, which, however, was not available in this location. If a talectomy is selected as treatment, it is preferable to perform this bilaterally so as to maintain equal limb length. Although it may be preferable to perform simultaneous bilateral talectomy, this decision always depends on the ability of the patient to manage non–weight bearing for a prolonged period of time. The family and social circumstances of the patient and their resources in planning this type of surgery have to be considered.

With the magnitude of this deformity, a talectomy may not be sufficient for correction of the hindfoot, and performing additional procedures in order to decompress the hindfoot has to be considered (**Fig. 1**A–C). Also, in **Fig. 1**C the contracture of the metatarsophalangeal (MP) joints, in particular, the hallux, can be seen. Generally, the flex contracture of the hallux corrects after bone decompression posteriorly but additional procedures on the toes to restore a neutral and mobile MP joint have to be anticipated. The authors have found that a transfibular approach to the talectomy is preferable to an approach anteriorly, which removes the talus piecemeal. After the lateral incision, the distal fibula is removed completely to expose the talus. There are 2 options for

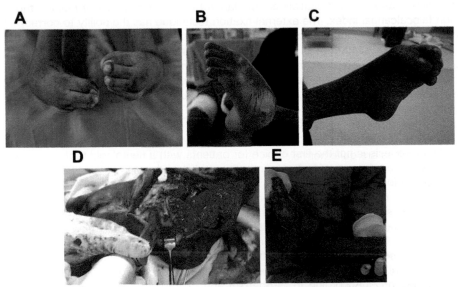

Fig. 1. (*A*) A 28-year-old woman presented with untreated bilateral club foot deformities. Both the feet (*B*) and the ankles (*C*) were in extremely rigid equinovarus. (*C*) The contracture of the MP joints, in particular, the hallux. (*D*) On the left foot, a transfibular approach to the talectomy was performed. In this case, after the talectomy, a very large lateral based wedge was removed at the level of the calcaneocuboid joint to address the residual adduction deformity through the transverse tarsal joint. (*E*) A very satisfactory correction of the deformity was achieved intraoperatively.

managing the fibula, 1 that includes discarding it, and, in the other procedure, the fibular is peeled back posteriorly, the talus removed, and then the fibula fixed with a plate to improve stability of the calcaneus in the ankle mortise. An osteotome is inserted into the ankle joint, which is gradually opened, and the talus slowly mobilized from its soft tissue attachments. It generally is easy to disarticulate the talus from the ankle joint but not as easy to remove it off the calcaneus until the interosseous ligament has been cut. In this case, after the talectomy, the hindfoot did not correct. There was persistent adduction deformity through the transverse tarsal joint, and further resection had to be performed at the level of the calcaneocuboid joint, where a very large wedge was removed (**Fig. 1D**). No attempt was made to perform an arthrodesis of the tibia to the calcaneus. The authors and other investigators, as discussed previously, have found that it generally is not necessary, and, provided the hindfoot is stable after immobilization, most patients tolerate this very well. It is believed that in talectomy cases, maintaining a correct position of the calcaneus is a key factor of the surgical outcome.[22,24,25]

At this stage, the most important aspect of the procedure is to ensure that there is adequate circulation to the foot. The tourniquet should be released routinely after bone removal before the foot is fixed in its final position. In this case, ischemia of the foot was present. In the presence of ischemia, the most important treatment is to wait and see what happens to the circulation after a few minutes leaving the foot hanging over the edge of the table. Warm moist sponges can be used, and, if the circulation still does not improve, a tunnel release must be performed. It is useful to have a Doppler ultrasound available to be able to map out the vessels, which may be compressed or twisted, in particular, the anterior tibial artery at the level of the ankle. The other alternative is to use nitroglycerin paste, which produces vasodilatation and may improve perfusion. The authors applied this paste liberally to the foot and 5 minutes later circulation had been restored completely. The final correction of the deformity intraoperatively is indicated in **Fig. 1E**.

RECURRENT CLUBFOOT

A recurrent clubfoot can develop either from failed serial stretching and casting treatment, including the Ponseti method, or from previous surgical treatment. Both surgeons and patients need to accept that due to complicated teratologic, neurologic, or even patients' personal circumstances, residual deformities and recurrence of the deformities are quite normal.[26] According to the literature, there is approximately 20% to 30% recurrence associated with idiopathic clubfoot, and 20% of clubfeet may require further surgical correction to address residual deformities even after a successful conservative treatment.[27] As long as the foot is asymptomatic, plantigrade, and functional, however, even with the assistance of orthotics or splints, no further surgical intervention is necessary. Revision surgery should be considered only to improve function and reduce symptoms.

Residual or recurrent deformities or even overcorrection may lead to equinus, varus, valgus, cavus, supination, and adduction. As with the mechanism of primary deformities of clubfeet, recurrent deformities usually are caused by soft tissue imbalance, which can be unbalanced muscle strength, static soft tissue contracture, or both. In the midfoot, the anterior tibial and the peroneal longus tendons keep the first ray in plantar flexion and dorsal flexion balance. The Achilles tendon and the anterior tibial tendon are a pair maintaining the foot in plantar flexion and dorsiflexion balance, and, with the posterior tibial tendon (PTT) and the peroneal brevis tendon, keep the foot in inversion and eversion balance. A relatively strong

Achilles tendon pulls the hindfoot into equinus if an Achilles tenotomy has not been done when it is necessary. Unbalanced relative strong posterior tibial and anterior tibial muscles force the foot into varus, whereas an overacting anterior tibial muscle drives the forefoot into adduction and the first ray into elevation. The secondary effect of this is to cause hallux rigidus with a plantar flexion contracture of the first MP joint, which also known is as a dorsal bunion. Plantar fascia contracture, a relatively strong peroneal longus muscle, and a weak anterior tibial muscle all can contribute to a midfoot cavus deformity. Vice versa, contracted soft tissue on the lateral side and a relatively tight or strong peroneal brevis from either an undercorrection or an overcorrection cause a valgus deformity in the midfoot or hindfoot.[26,28–31] Therefore, the need to address any potential static or dynamic soft tissue imbalance with soft tissue releases and tendon transfers, where necessary, always should be borne in mind. Claw toes usually are caused by soft tissue imbalance either from the primary deformity, which includes weakness of the intrinsic muscles, dysfunctional anterior tibial muscle, and overaction of the extensor longus muscles, with contracture of the plantar fascia and extensor brevis muscles, and flexor muscles, or from a corrective surgery of the hindfoot. As is known, in bringing the ankle from an equinus contracture to the neutral position, the flexor tendons are put under greater tension, which can cause a claw toe deformity. For a primary claw toe deformity, treatment options include tenotomy of the extensor brevis tendons, lengthening of the longus extensor tendons, excision of the flexor longus tendons, release of dorsal and lateral soft tissue of the MP joint, and arthroplasty or arthrodesis of the proximal phalangeal joint. The approach to correction depends on the flexibility of the toe, which should be reassessed after each step. For a secondary claw toe deformity, which is caused by correction of a severe equinus ankle, the treatment may be postponed as a staged surgery to avoid ischemic complications, particularly in cases where extensive bony and soft tissue procedures already have been done in the midfoot and hindfoot. With severe equinus, as the foot is brought up to a neutral position, both the short and long flexors are contracted. It is easy to correct the contracture of the long flexors with tenotomy but not the short flexors. These may elongate slightly after the plantar fascia release but may remain contracted, limiting dorsiflexion of the MP joints. This is difficult to treat, and the only way to increase dorsiflexion is to either remove the metatarsal heads in severe cases or shorten the metatarsal with a distal osteotomy to relieve the flexion contracture.

The authors present a 23-year-old patient who had been treated for a club foot deformity during early childhood and operated on twice with recurrence of deformity. Note the severity of the unilateral deformity, which was not entirely rigid (**Fig. 2**A, B). Intraoperatively, the foot was examined and noted to have mobility in the ankle, albeit slightly limited due to a flat top talus. Limited correction of this deformity with manipulation (**Fig. 2**C, D) can be appreciated. Based on the mobility of the ankle, it was decided to preserve the ankle joint and perform only a triple arthrodesis with a medial soft tissue releases, including a percutaneous posterior tibial tenotomy with incision of the spring ligament, which made the foot slightly more mobile. The rest of the procedure was performed through an extensile lateral incision. Commencing with the subtalar joint, a lateral wedge was removed from the joint using a sharp osteotome until the hindfoot could be corrected into slight valgus (**Fig. 2**E, F). The majority of the correction was performed through the transverse tarsal joint by resecting a large biplanar wedge commencing at the calcaneocuboid joint and entering into the talonavicular joint. The first cut was made on the calcaneus and talus (**Fig. 2**G), followed by removal of a larger wedge from the cuboid and navicular (**Fig. 2**H). At the completion of the joint

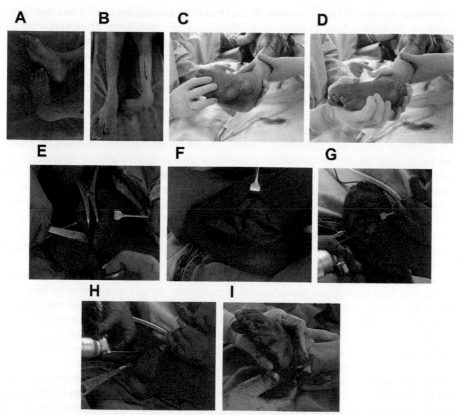

Fig. 2. A 23-year-old patient had been operated for a clubfoot deformity in her left foot during early childhood. (*A*) Note the recurrence of the deformity in the left foot (*B*). Although the deformity was severe (*C*), there was some mobility in the ankle and the foot and limited correction could be achieved with manipulation (*D*). A triple arthrodesis with medial soft tissue releases was planned. In performing the triple arthrodesis, a large biplanar wedge on both the lateral and dorsal sides was resected (*E*) through the transverse tarsal joint in order to correct the majority of the deformity (*F*). The first cut was made on the calcaneus and talus (*G*), followed by removal of a larger wedge from the cuboid and navicular (*H*). Note the neutral hindfoot position after removing the biplanar wedge (*I*).

preparation, the foot easily could be manipulated into a neutral hindfoot position (**Fig. 2I**). Further work was performed on the toes, which were contracted preoperatively and slightly more so after the hindfoot correction.

CALCANEOVALGUS

Congenital calcaneovalgus deformity, also known as reverse clubfoot,[32,33] is a type of deformity that is seen far less commonly than equinovarus. According to a study of the Edinburgh Register of the Newborn 1964 to 1968, including 52,029 births in the city during the 4.5 years, there were only 22 cases of talipes calcaneovalgus.[34] The congenital calcaneovalgus deformity, which must be differentiated from a congenital vertical talus,[35,36] is characterized by calcaneus at the ankle and valgus at the subtalar joint.[32,35–38] Dislocation of the peroneal tendons on the lateral side and contracture of the Achilles tendon posteriorly and anterior tibial tendon anteriorly have been considered as part of both the etiology and result of the deformity.[38] The Edinburgh Newborn Register study showed that there was an incidence of developmental dysplasia of the hip of 0.6%.[34] Westberry and colleagues[39] reported an incidence of 0.28% of developmental dysplasia of the hip with congenital talipes calcaneovalgus. Paton and Choudry's[40] 11-year prospective longitudinal observational study of the relationship between neonatal deformities of the foot and the presence of ultrasonographic developmental dysplasia of the hip showed an overall risk of 1:5.2 of ultrasonographic dysplasia or instability in congenital talipes calcaneovalgus. Muscle imbalance caused by muscular neurologic disorders, such as spina bifida, polio, and cerebral palsy, are additional causes of calcaneovalgus deformities.[41] There can be a wide variety of combined congenital and acquired deformities, such as contracture or dislocation of the hip, contracture or valgus/varus deformities of the knee, and rotation of lower limbs. In those circumstances, treating the proximal deformities of the limb other than focusing only on the foot and ankle and balancing the lower limb muscle strength are the key points for a satisfactory outcome.[42] Treatment includes early splinting and serial casting for primary flexible deformities[32] and surgeries for severe, rigid, or residual deformities and deformities with muscle strength imbalance.[43]

The authors present a severely disabled 15-year old child, who was unable to wear shoes. She had a profound calcaneovalgus deformity, which was markedly unstable (**Fig. 3**A). The foot could be dislocated and was extremely unstable at the level of the ankle (**Fig. 3**B), most likely due to a ball-and-socket ankle. The foot could be straightened with manipulation (**Fig. 3**C) but the peroneal tendons and Achilles tendon were extremely contracted. With the hindfoot held in a relatively neutral position, the forefoot was markedly supinated with instability present in the midfoot.

This child had difficulty ambulating, and an ideal goal for her was simultaneous bilateral correction. Despite her age, she weighed very little, and her mother felt that she would be able to cope with lifting her and moving her around the home. Therefore, bilateral surgery was performed. There were many procedures that could be considered for correction, but, due to the profound instability as well as the contraction posterolaterally, a tibiotalocalcaneal (TTC) arthrodesis was chosen, despite her age. The procedure was performed through a lateral incision and a transfibular approach used to address both the ankle and subtalar joints. A tenotomy of the Achilles tendon and peroneal tendons then were performed. When performing an Achilles tenotomy, the authors recommend that the incision is made from the inside rather than percutaneously to avoid gapping of the skin after correction.

The authors find that it is easier to begin with the subtalar joint while the ankle joint is still relatively stable. At this age, the articular surface can be scraped using a fine osteotome; however, care must be taken not to remove more of the articular surface laterally in either the subtalar or ankle joint, which would produce a valgus malunion. The ankle then is dislocated medially so that the entire articular surface is visible. This makes it easier to make the surface preparation of the ankle joint and identify the source of instability (**Fig. 3**D). The joint can be prepared either using a sharp osteotome or, in this case, using a fine saw to cut the joint surface, as seen in **Fig. 3**E.

Fixation of the TTC arthrodesis was straightforward, using 2.5-mm pins. In **Fig. 3**F, the hindfoot is well aligned with respect to the tibia but there is marked forefoot supination present. This likely was the result of a contracture of the anterior tibial tendon, which was now unmasked as a result of correction of the hindfoot. In addition to the supination of the forefoot, there also was abduction instability noted in the midfoot, and a closing wedge arthrodesis of the naviculocuneiform joints also was performed. The final appearance of the foot with the midfoot arthrodesis and the lateral transfer of

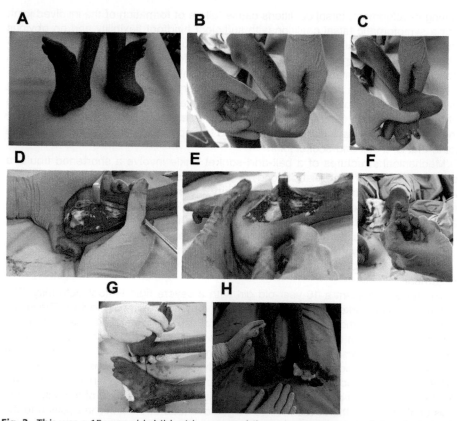

Fig. 3. This was a 15-year-old child with a severe bilateral calcaneovalgus deformity in both ankles (*A*). The ankles were extremely unstable and could be dislocated easily into dorsal calcaneovalgus (*B*) and partially straightened with manipulation (*C*). Due to the profound instability and the severe posterior contraction, a TTC arthrodesis was performed through a lateral transfibular approach. The subtalar joint was prepared first and then the talus was dislocated medially to expose the whole ankle joint (*D*). Then ankle joint surface was cut using a fine saw (*E*). Note the hindfoot was well aligned according to the tibia after the TTC procedure, but there was obvious forefoot supination (*F*), which was corrected by closing wedge arthrodesis of the naviculocuneiform joints and an anterior tibial tendon lateral transfer (*G*). The transferred anterior tibial tendon was fixed onto the plantar surface of the foot using the rubber stopper from a 20-mL syringe as a type of suture button (*H*).

the anterior tibial tendon are shown in **Fig. 3**G. Fixation of the anterior tibial tendon transfer was performed using a rubber stopper taken from a 20-mL syringe. The syringe is taken apart, and the rubber stopper is removed and perforated with a small hemostat clamp through which the 2 sutures from the tendon are now passed. The rubber stopper then is used as a type of button over thick gauze padding on the plantar surface of the foot. The authors find that this is much safer than using a button because it is less rigid and less likely to cause skin necrosis (**Fig. 3**H).

TARSAL COALITION BALL-AND-SOCKET ANKLE JOINT

Tarsal coalitions include talocalcaneal, calcaneonavicular, and, less commonly, the talonavicular joint. As a result of failure of segmentation of the primitive mesenchyme during development, tarsal coalitions cause failure of formation of the involved joint. For a symptomatic tarsal coalition with sufficient hindfoot flexibility and no obvious degeneration of adjacent joints, a coalition resection with other supplementary procedures usually are performed to restore the hindfoot alignment and stability, such as a medial displacement calcaneal osteotomy, a calcaneus stop procedure, or a cotton osteotomy. For a tarsal coalition case with a very rigid hindfoot or significant joint arthritis, a subtalar joint fusion or a double or triple arthrodesis is used. Due to the abnormal restriction of motion in the foot from an early age, more severe coalitions, in particular the talonavicular, sometimes lead to a spherical malformation of the ankle joint, that is, a ball-and-socket joint.[44,45]

Mechanical structures of a ball-and-socket ankle involve a shortened fibula, a spherical shape of the tibial plafond, and a valgus ankle and hindfoot deformity. All of these plus increased hindfoot rigidity caused by the tarsal coalition lead to decreased ankle stability.[46] For a ball-and-socket ankle presenting in a young age or even in adults without evidence of ankle arthritis, a supramalleolar osteotomy can be performed to restore the shape of the ankle. Although, for an adult patient with advanced arthritis of the ankle due to long-term uneven loading and instability of the joint, an ankle arthrodesis is a more appropriate treatment.[46,47]

The authors present a 16-year-old girl with a severe rigid flatfoot deformity. The hindfoot was in marked valgus, and there was extreme rigidity of the foot. The ankle, however, was very mobile, indicating the possibility of ankle instability associated with that ball-and-socket ankle (**Fig. 4**A, B). Radiographs and a CT scan confirmed the presence of the tarsal coalition and a severe deformity of the talonavicular joint (**Fig. 4**C–F). The CT scan of the ankle was highly unusual, with a varus ankle deformity in the presence of such severe hindfoot valgus. In addition, there were cystic changes on the lateral aspect of the distal tibia, indicating a lateral overload of the ankle joint. This confirmed that there was marked valgus overload of the ankle in addition to the valgus deformity of the hindfoot.

Given the severity of the valgus deformity all of the ankle joint, a medial closing wedge supramalleolar osteotomy was performed first (**Fig. 4**G). It is important when performing this osteotomy that it is planned according to the size of the plate that is to be used for fixation, which should be approximately 4 cm proximal to the tibiotalar joint surface. In a situation like this, it rarely is necessary to perform a simultaneous fibular osteotomy. A small wedge should be commenced with and then slightly more bone removed as needed until the ankle is in a neutral position (**Fig. 4**H). At the completion of the tibial osteotomy, the ankle was well aligned and planning of the hindfoot correction can be begun. Due to the severity of the deformity, a medial approach to correction was planned by performing a medial double arthrodesis (talonavicular and subtalar joints). Prior to commencing with the arthrodesis, a percutaneous tenotomy of the peroneus brevis was performed laterally (**Fig. 4**I). Without this, it is unlikely that the severe valgus deformity could be corrected. The approach to the subtalar and talonavicular joints began with exposure of the flexor tendons. By retracting the flexor digitorum longus dorsally and the flexor hallucis longus (FHL) inferiorly, the subtalar joint can be identified, simultaneously protecting the neurovascular bundle behind the FHL (**Fig. 4**J). The authors found that it was not necessary to completely expose the entire subtalar joint. Although the subtalar joint was exposed and débrided, the bone cut was made through the calcaneus as close to the joint as possible in order to medially translate the tuberosity (**Fig. 4**K). A small biplanar wedge was removed from the talonavicular joint, permitting adduction and slight plantar flexion of the foot through the talonavicular joint (**Fig. 4**L). The intraoperative

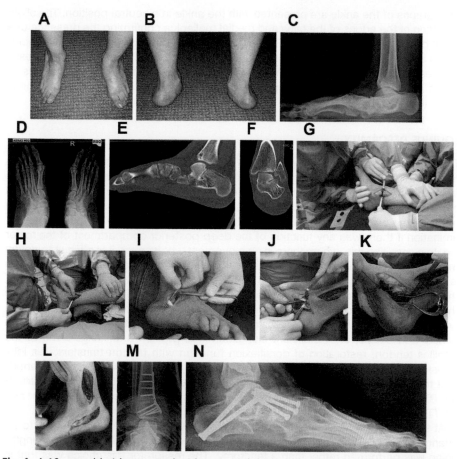

Fig. 4. A 16-year-old girl presented with a severe bilateral rigid flatfoot deformity. Note the profound bilateral hindfoot valgus both from the anterior (A) and posterior views (B). A decision to treat the right foot first was made. Lateral (C) and anteroposterior (D) radiographs, and sagittal (E) and coronal (F) plane CT scan showed the presence of a tarsal coalition and a severe deformity of the talonavicular joint. A medial closing wedge supramalleolar osteotomy was performed first to correct the marked valgus deformity of the ankle joint (G) and a plate applied (H). To correct the hindfoot valgus, a percutaneous tenotomy of the peroneus brevis was performed laterally (I), and then a double arthrodesis of the talonavicular and subtalar joints was done through a medial approach. While doing the subtalar joint arthrodesis through a medial approach, by retracting the FDL dorsally and the FHL inferiorly (J), the subtalar joint can be identified easily with protecting the neurovascular bundle behind the FHL (K). A small biplanar wedge was removed from the talonavicular joint permitting adduction and slight plantar flexion of the foot through the talonavicular joint (L). Intraoperative radiographs showed the ankle was in a neutral positions (M). The slight rounding of the edges of the talus and medial malleolus can be appreciated, confirming the presence of a slight ball-and-socket ankle joint (M). The final lateral radiograph at 8 weeks after surgery showed very good correction, arthrodesis, and restoration of the arch. Note the markedly improved talar declination angle as well as the calcaneal pitch angle (N).

radiographs of the ankle are presented with the ankle in a neutral position. The slight rounding of the edges of the talus and medial malleolus confirming the presence of a slight ball-and-socket ankle joint (**Fig. 4**M) can be appreciated. The final lateral radiograph at 8 weeks after surgery is presented, noting very good correction, arthrodesis, and restoration of the arch. Note the plantar translation of the calcaneus tuberosity, which markedly improved the talar declination angle as well as the calcaneal pitch angle (**Fig. 4**N).

EQUINUS DEFORMITY

The patient in **Fig. 5** was a young man who suffered a knee injury and a complete peroneal nerve palsy with a resulting foot drop and eventual fixed contracture of the entire foot 6 months later. The authors had the opportunity to treat him 9 months after his injury and he was unable to ambulate, stand, or wear a shoe (**Fig. 5**A, B). On examination, there was no movement in the ankle whatsoever, and it was not clear on examination if there was any function of the deep posterior compartment of the lower leg. In a case like this, where there is no movement whatsoever, it is difficult to determine if there is any function of the posterior tibial muscle or if the tendon and or muscle is scarred. In other circumstances, an MRI of the leg may be able to be obtained and the muscle evaluated for fatty infiltration and atrophy, but these were not possible in this location. Therefore, the authors had to anticipate numerous alternative procedures for correction, which would include a TTC arthrodesis, a talectomy and tibiocalcaneal arthrodesis, or, if sufficient elongation was present after lengthening of the Achilles tendon, restoration of dorsiflexion function with tendon transfers. If a PTT transfer were performed, it could function either as a dynamic transfer or as a tenodesis to maintain the position of the foot. In this case, ultimately there was mobility of the PTT and it had to be assumed that some muscle function would be present and a PTT transfer through the interosseous membrane was performed.

At surgery, a posterolateral incision was used, which was versatile enough to be changed to any of the procedures discussed previously. An Achilles tendon lengthening was performed rather than a tenotomy. The reason for this choice was that in the event that a neutral foot was attained, after a PTT transfer to the dorsum of the foot, overactivity of dorsiflexion could occur and, in the presence of an absent gastrocnemius, it would cause a calcaneus deformity. It was not necessary to perform a posterior ankle capsulotomy. After the Achilles tendon release, however, a neutral foot was attained, which produced severe contractures of the hallux and lesser toes, as seen in **Fig. 5**C. The contractures were only in the long flexor tendons and not associated with contractures of the MP joints, that is, the short flexors and intrinsic muscles. Therefore, simple tenotomies of the tendons were performed percutaneously under the interphalangeal joints. Once a neutral foot had been obtained, mobility of the PTT was checked. There was no scarring of the tendon and some mobility was noted, and the authors assumed that some muscle function remained, but as discussed previously, it was difficult to determine preoperatively. A PTT transfer then was performed through the interosseous membrane (**Fig. 5**D). Despite the flexor tenotomies, there was still a slight lag at the MP joints as a result of the weakness of the toe extensor muscles. For this reason, a transfer of all of the long toe extensors (a Hibbs procedure) was performed to the midfoot (**Fig. 5**E) but only to serve as a tenodesis to help prevent the toes from dropping in flexion. The outcome of the procedure can be seen in **Figs. 5**F and 5G at 6 weeks after the surgery, and the patient was walking at 3 months with a plantigrade foot and managing well without a brace (**Fig. 5**H).

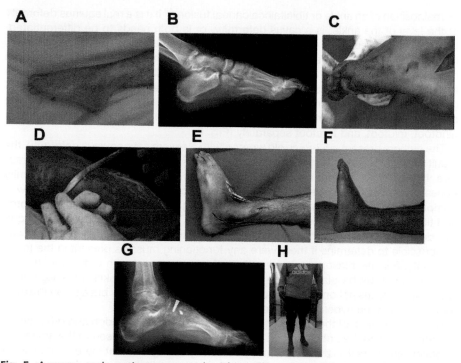

Fig. 5. A young male patient presented with a stiff equinus deformity in his left foot 9 months after a knee injury, which had caused complete peroneal nerve palsy. Both clinical (*A*) and radiographic (*B*) examinations showed severe equinus deformity at the ankle level. An Achilles tendon lengthening was performed. After the ankle was corrected into neutral position, severe contractures of the hallux and lesser toes presented (*C*) due to passive tightening of the long flexor tendons. Therefore, simple tenotomies of the long flexor tendons were performed. Then the PTT was transferred laterally through the interosseous membrane on to the lateral cuneiform (*D*). A Hibbs procedure was used to transfer all of the long toe extensor tendons to the midfoot to serve as a tenodesis to help prevent the toes from dropping in flexion (*E*). Note the clinical (*F*) and radiographic (*G*) outcome of the treatment at 6 weeks after the surgery, and the patient walking with a plantigrade foot without a brace at 3 months after the surgery (*H*).

Note the difference between an active tendon transfer and a tenodesis procedure. An active tendon transfer is used when there is sufficient muscle strength to use which is at least grade 4, so that the tendon can be placed in a new location to strengthen the weak/dysfunction muscle. Moreover, this is also based on the flexibility of the involved joint(s). In the presence of a flaccid paralysis of the limb, where the muscle function is not present, the authors can use the muscle and the tendon as a static sling structure by doing a tenodesis to help with maintaining a plantigrade foot. Although in the long run a tenodesis may fail due to stretching, it does have some role of preventing a drop foot.

CAVOEQUINUS

Equinus deformity refers to excessive fixed plantarflexion of the ankle beyond a neutral position and can be caused by a weak anterior tibial muscle, bony factors such as a vertical talus, or overactive triceps surae or for iatrogenic reasons, such as malposition of an ankle or tibialtalocalcaneal fusion.[48] If it is a real equinus deformity at the level of the ankle, is a cavus deformity, or is both needs to be differentiated, because the equinus may exist only in the forefoot with a neutral hindfoot and ankle, for example, after a TTC arthrodesis. Lateral radiographs of the ankle and foot are more helpful in diagnosis than judging only from physical examination because the apex of the deformity rarely can be appreciated clinically. Sometimes even radiographs, however, also are misleading. One way to determine the apex of the deformity and differentiate a cavus from an equinus is to evaluate the deformity by covering the hindfoot, midfoot, and forefoot separately (**Fig. 6**).

The authors present a 52-year-old woman with a severe cavoequinus deformity, the result of poliomyelitis. The predominant deformity is of course the equinus contracture, but a severe midfoot cavus also is present (**Fig. 7**A–D). This type of deformity poses significant challenges for planning correction. The equinus contracture was completely rigid, and the possibility of performing a TTC arthrodesis, a talectomy and tibiocalcaneal arthrodesis, or other procedures as necessary to correct the equinus deformity had to be anticipated. Due to the magnitude of the contracture, it was not possible to determine if there were any functioning muscles present in the lower extremity. For this reason, combining the ankle realignment with a dynamic tendon transfer could not be planned. The goal, therefore, had to be skeletal realignment, which had to focus not only on correction of the equinus deformity but also on the midfoot cavus and the hyperextension of the toe MP joints.

Because position of the foot after tenotomy of the Achilles tendon and other flexor tendons could not be anticipated, a transfibular approach was used to the ankle and subtalar joint as well as the soft tissues posteriorly. In **Fig. 7**E, that there is no incision posteriorly over the Achilles tendon. This is consistent with the authors' approach for managing severe equinus deformity with the tendon cut from inside to avoid any gapping of the skin with correction of the deformity. After the Achilles tenotomy,

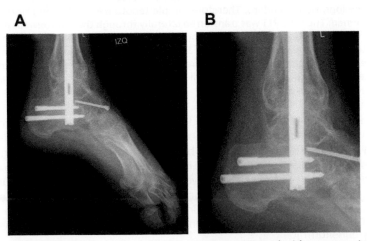

Fig. 6. Case from Concepción, Chile. A 31-year-old man presented with a cavoequinus deformity in his left foot with a previous TTC plus a talonavicular fusion. On the lateral radiographic view of the foot, by covering the midfoot and forefoot from the previous talonavicular joint, the problem was a cavus deformity in the talonavicular and naviculocuneiform joints instead of an equinus deformity in the ankle (A). Therefore, for this case, a revision with a midfoot dorsal wedge arthrodesis through the talonavicular and naviculocuneiform joints is sufficient to address the deformity (B).

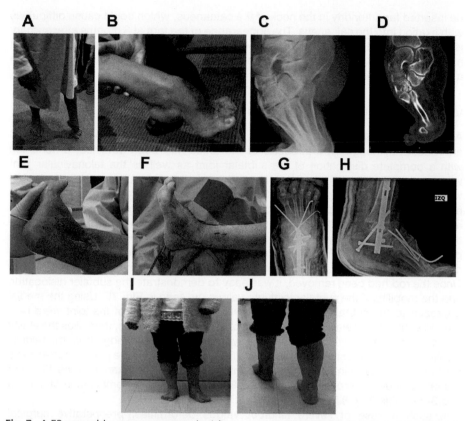

Fig. 7. A 52-year-old woman presented with a severe cavoequinus deformity in her left foot as a result of poliomyelitis (*A*), with severe midfoot cavus on both clinical examination (*B*), radiograph imaging (*C*), and CT scan (*D*). An Achilles tendon tenotomy was performed through the same transfibular approach, which was used later for a TTC fusion (*E*). Percutaneous tenotomy of the peroneal tendons, PTT, FHL, and FDL, and a midfoot wedge osteotomy were performed to correct both the hindfoot and midfoot deformities. Note the final clinical appearance of the foot (*F*). Note that on the radiographs, the talus was intentionally translated anteriorly in order for the intramedullary rod to purchase the bodies of the talus (*G*) and the calcaneus (*H*). Note the appearance of the foot at 3 months after surgery from the front (*I*) and back while walking (*J*).).

the remaining tendons, including the peroneals, posterior tibial, FHL, and flexor digitorum longus, were cut percutaneously. The subtalar joint was prepared using a sharp osteotome, and the ankle joint using a saw followed by realignment of the hind foot and ankle and intramedullary fixation. This corrected the equinus deformity very well, but the midfoot cavus remained, and this was addressed using an anterior and central incision over the midfoot, where a midfoot wedge was removed from the navicular cuneiform joint. The final clinical appearance of the foot is indicated in **Fig. 7**F. It is curious that in this case, after correction of the deformity, there was no significant contracture of the flexor tendons causing a fixed claw toe deformity. This most likely was due to the hyperextension that existed preoperatively from chronic weight bearing on the forefoot with hyperextension of the MP joints. On the radiographs (**Fig. 7**G, H), the talus has been intentionally translated anteriorly. If the talus had been centered directly under the tibia, the intramedullary rod would be inserted far anteriorly in the neck of the calcaneus, which could cause difficulties with fixation into the calcaneus. The appearance of the foot at 3 months after surgery is shown in **Fig. 7**I and J. She had a stable arthrodesis of both the hindfoot ankle and midfoot, had very nicely aligned toes, and was able to ambulate quite comfortably in a shoe, here barefoot.

VALGUS DISLOCATION OF THE HINDFOOT

A 62-year-old patient with rheumatoid arthritis had previously undergone a TTC arthrodesis. Although an arthrodesis of the ankle had been obtained, a nonunion with a complete dislocation of the subtalar joint as well as the talonavicular joint was present (**Fig. 8A**, B). The rod was protruding inferiorly and the patient bearing weight on the medial aspect of the foot, which was extremely painful. The foot was markedly deformed and fairly rigid (**Fig. 8C**). The decision making was how to approach restoration of the alignment of the foot given the rigidity of the deformity, the condition of the skin medially and laterally, and the potential for wound-healing problems if a lateral approach was used. A decision, therefore, was made to use an all medial approach to correction of the deformity, as demonstrated in **Fig. 8D**. Once the rod had been removed, it was easy to demonstrate the subtalar dislocation and the mobility of the subtalar joint into valgus, as seen in **Fig. 7E**. Using the medial approach to the subtalar joint, débridement and preparation of the joint were performed until the heel was in a neutral position (**Fig. 8F**). From here, there was the ability to focus on the talonavicular dislocation by removing a large wedge from the talonavicular joint medially using a saw (**Fig. 8G**). The foot was now quite plantigrade and in a neutral position both in the hindfoot and midfoot (**Fig. 8H**, I). Fixation of the TTC and the talonavicular arthrodesis was accomplished the use of a combination of screws and 3-mm pins (**Fig. 8J**).

In such a case of severe hindfoot valgus deformities, preoperative surgical approach planning to get access to subtalar joint is critical to the success of the surgery. Surgeons must realize that the conventional lateral approach limits the capability of deformity correction and can add the risk of wound-healing problems. Using the single medial approach is a much safer and an easier option for preparing both the subtalar joint and the talonavicular joint and taking out a medially based wedge in order to correct severe midfoot abduction.[49–53] According to extensive literature reports, the medial approach has been used successfully in patients with high risk of wound complications, such as diabetes, rheumatoid arthritis, a severe deformity with contracted lateral skin, and soft tissue.[54–56]

Concerns with regard to the single medial approach for double or triple arthrodesis include the ability of exposing the subtalar joints, the union rate, possible risk of medial tendons and ligaments injury, vascular disruption of the talus and subsequent talar osteonecrosis, and so forth. Widnall and colleagues[57] modified the approach described previously by Jeng and colleagues.[51] Through an incision parallel to and just above the PTT running from just posterior to the medial malleolus to just distal to the navicular bone, using the sustentaculum tali as a bony landmark, access to both the middle and the posterior facets of the subtalar joint and the talonavicular joint could be achieved with retention of the PTT, the tibiocalcaneal ligament, and the spring ligament. A cadaveric study demonstrated that the medial neurovascular bundle was 21 mm from the medial approach.[58,59] Another cadaveric investigation found that both the single medial incision approach and the traditional 2-incision approach could result in substantial disruption of the main blood supply to the talus. Necrosis of the talus has not been reported, however, in medial incision–approached

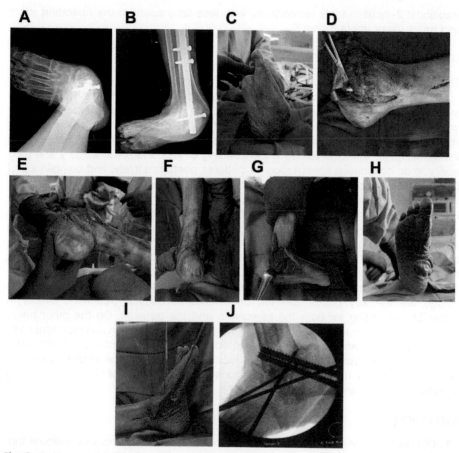

Fig. 8. A 62-year-old patient with rheumatoid arthritis presented with a nonunion with a complete dislocation of the talonavicular joint (A) as well as the subtalar joint (B) after an attempted previous TTC arthrodesis. Note the rod was protruding inferiorly (B). The foot was markedly deformed, and fairly rigid (C). Given the rigidity of the deformity and the potential for wound-healing problems, if a lateral approach was used, an all medial approach was chosen to correct the deformity (D). Using the medial approach to the subtalar joint (E), the débridement and preparation of the joint were performed until the heel was in a neutral position (F). Then, the talonavicular dislocation was addressed by removing a large wedge medially using a saw (G). The foot was now quite plantigrade (H), and in a neutral position both in the hindfoot and midfoot (I). Fixation was accomplished by the use of a combination of screws and 3-mm pins (J).

hindfoot fusion.[60] Jeng and colleagues[50] reported that in performing a triple arthrodesis through the single medial incision, more than 90% of both subtalar and talonavicular joints could be prepared, and even 90% of the calcaneocuboid joint also could be accessed, which was comparable to the standard 2-incision approach for a triple arthrodesis. According to Brilhault's[55] cohort study in 14 feet with very high risk of lateral wound breakdown, at an average of 20 months' follow-up, the investigators had found significant radiographic correction and no wound complications. The literature also reported comparable union rate[52,60] and deformity correction capability[61] of the double arthrodesis through a medial approach to a traditional 2-incision triple arthrodesis, with less time spent in the operating room and much lower implant cost.[61]

SUMMARY

The severe foot and ankle deformities that the authors' organization has encountered in different humanitarian programs worldwide are much more complicated than those surgeons treat in their daily practice in developed countries. In a humanitarian program, various factors, including the severity of the deformity, the patients' economic limitations, patients' expectations and realistic needs in life, availability of surgical instrumentation, the local team's understanding of foot and ankle surgery and their ability to do continuous consultation for patients postoperatively, and compliance of the patients all account for the success of the surgery. Detailed communication with the local orthopedic team, patients and their families, and within the medical care delivery team is critical. Because most of the surgeon volunteers themselves are from many parts of the world, however, the huge cultural differences between the surgeons and the patients always make the surgery more challenging than just a deformity correction. Under these circumstances, following basic rules of deformity correction, such as always addressing both soft tissue imbalance and bony malalignment whenever necessary and choosing classic surgeries, such as arthrodesis with high reliability, are the key points. On the one hand, successful treatment always is incredibly rewarding for both the caregivers and the patients. On the other hand, regardless of how much effort surgeons have made, complications and recurrence still occur, in particular among the patients treated when essential continuous follow-up is limited for various reasons. Therefore, educating and training the local surgeons to take over the future medical care are the most important goals of the authors' global humanitarian programs.

REFERENCES

1. Dhillon MS, Sandhu HS. Surgical options in the management of residual foot problems in poliomyelitis. Foot Ankle Clin 2000;5(2):327–47.
2. Myerson MS, Kadakia AR. Reconstructive foot and ankle surgery: management of complications. 3rd edition. Philadelphia: Elsevier; 2018.
3. Albright RH, Waverly BJ, Klein E, et al. Percutaneous Kirschner wire versus commercial implant for hammertoe repair: a cost-effectiveness analysis. J Foot Ankle Surg 2018;57(2):332–8.
4. Karlock LG, Berry L, Craft ST, et al. First metatarsophalangeal joint fusion with use of crossed Kirschner wires and intramedullary Steinmann pin. J Foot Ankle Surg 2017;56(6):1139–42.
5. Roye DP Jr, Roye BD. Idiopathic congenital talipes equinovarus. J Am Acad Orthop Surg 2002;10(4):239–48.
6. Grant AD, Atar D, Lehman WB. The Ilizarov technique in correction of complex foot deformities. Clin Orthop Relat Res 1992;280:94–103.
7. Ferreira RC, Costo MT, Frizzo GG, et al. Correction of neglected clubfoot using the Ilizarov external fixator. Foot Ankle Int 2006;27(4):266–73.
8. Hernigou P, Huys M, Pariat J, et al. History of clubfoot treatment, part I: from manipulation in antiquity to splint and plaster in Renaissance before tenotomy. Int Orthop 2017;41(8):1693–704.
9. Beals RK. Club foot in the Maori: a genetic study of 50 kindreds. N Z Med J 1978; 88(618):144–6.

10. Culverwell AD, Tapping CR. Congenital talipes equinovarus in Papua New Guinea: a difficult yet potentially manageable situation. Int Orthop 2009;33(2): 521–6.
11. Coleman S. Teratologic equinovarus congenita. In: Coleman S, editor. Complex foot deformities in children. Philadelphia: Lea & Feibger; 1983. p. 255–64.
12. van Wijick SF, Oomen AM, van der Heide HJ. Feasibility and barriers of treating clubfeet in four countries. Int Orthop 2015;39(12):2415–22.
13. Choi IH, Yang MS, Chung CY, et al. The treatment of recurrent arthrogrypotic club foot in children by the Ilizarov method. A preliminary report. J Bone Joint Surg Br 2001;83(5):731–7.
14. Menelaus MB. Talectomy for equinovarus deformity in arthrogryposis and spina bifida. J Bone Joint Surg Br 1971;53(3):468–73.
15. El-Sherbini MH, Omran AA. Midterm follow-up of talectomy for severe rigid equinovarus feet. J Foot Ankle Surg 2015;54(6):1093–8.
16. Ghali NN, Smith RB, Clayden AD, et al. The results of pantalar reduction in the management of congenital talipes equinovarus. J Bone Joint Surg Br 1983; 65(1):1–7.
17. Kocaoğlu M, Eralp L, Atalar AC, et al. Correction of complex foot deformities using the Ilizarov external fixator. J Foot Ankle Surg 2002;41(1):30–9.
18. Lee DY, Choi IH, Yoo WJ, et al. Application of the Ilizarov technique to the correction of neurologic equinocavovarus foot deformity. Clin Orthop Relat Res 2011; 469(3):860–7.
19. Guidera KJ, Drennan JC. Foot and ankle deformities in arthrogryposis multiplex congenita. Clin Orthop Relat Res 1985;194:93–8.
20. Saltzman CL, Fehrle MJ, Cooper RR, et al. Triple arthrodesis: twenty-five and forty-four-year average follow-up of the same patients. J Bone Joint Surg Am 1999;81(10):1391–402.
21. Lindseth RE. Myelomeningocele. In: Morrissy RT, Weinstein SL, editors. Philadelphia: Lippincott Williams & Wilkins; 2001.
22. Cooper RR, Talectomy CW. A long-term follow-up evaluation. Clin Orthop Relat Res 1985;201:32–5.
23. Zuccon A, Cardoso SI, Abreu FP, et al. Surgical treatment for myelodysplastic clubfoot. Rev Bras Ortop 2014;49(6):653–60.
24. Joseph TN, Myerson MS. Use of talectomy in modern foot and ankle surgery. Foot Ankle Clin 2004;9(4):775–85.
25. Dias LS, Stern LS. Talectomy in the treatment of resistant talipes equinovarus deformity in myelomeningocele and arthrogryposis. J Pediatr Orthop 1987;7(1): 39–41.
26. Uglow MG, Kurup HV. Residual clubfoot in children. Foot Ankle Clin N Am 2010; 15:245–64.
27. Docquier PL, Leemrijse T, Rombouts JJ. Clinical and radiographic features of operatively treated stiff clubfeet after skeletal maturity: etiology of the deformities and how to prevent them. Foot Ankle Int 2006;27(1):29–37.
28. Mosca VS. The cavus foot. J Pediatr Orthop 2001;21(4):423–4.
29. Thompson GH, Hoyen HA, Barthel T. Tibialis anterior tendon transfer after clubfoot surgery. Clin Orthop Relat Res 2009;467(5):1306–13.
30. Otremski I, Salama R, Khermosh O, et al. Residual adduction of the forefoot. A review of the Turco procedure for congenital club foot. J Bone Joint Surg Br 1987;69(5):832–4.

31. Haslam PG, Goddard M, Flowers MJ, et al. Overcorrection and generalized joint laxity in surgically treated congenital talipes equino-varus. J Pediatr Orthop B 2006;15(4):273–7.

32. Ferciot CF. Calcaneovalgus foot in the newborn and its relation to developmental flatfoot. Clin Orthop 1953;1:22–7.

33. Giannestras NJ. Dural and intradural compression as a cause of clubfoot. Clin Orthop 1953;1:28–32.

34. Wynne-Davies R, Littlejohn A, Gormley J. Aetiology and interrelationship of some common skeletal deformities. (Talipes equinovarus and calcaneovalgus, metatarsus varus, congenital dislocation of the hip, and infantile idiopathic scoliosis). J Med Genet 1982;19(5):321–8.

35. Brand RA. Dural and intradural compression as a cause of clubfoot. NJ Giannestras MD CORR 1953;1:28-32. Calcaneovalgus foot in the newborn and its relationship to development flatfoot. CF Ferciot MD CORR 1953;1:22-27. Clin Orthop Relat Res 2009;467(5):1385–6.

36. Hernigou P. History of clubfoot treatment; part III (twentieth century): back to the future. Int Orthop 2017;41(11):2407–14.

37. Yu GV, Hladik J. Residual calcaneovalgus deformity: review of the literature and case study. J Foot Ankle Surg 1994;33(3):228–38.

38. Edwards ER, Menelaus MB. Reverse club foot. Rigid and recalcitrant talipes calcaneovalgus. J Bone Joint Surg Br 1987;69(2):330–4.

39. Westberry DE, Davids JR, Pugh LI. Clubfoot and developmental dysplasia of the hip: value of screening hip radiographs in children with clubfoot. J Pediatr Orthop 2003;23(4):503–7.

40. Paton RW, Choudry Q. Neonatal foot deformities and their relationship to developmental dysplasia of the hip. J Bone Joint Surg Br 2009;91(5):655–8.

41. Faraj AA. Review of Elmslie's triple arthrodesis for post-polio pes calcaneovalgus deformity. J Foot Ankle Surg 1995;34(3):319–21.

42. Swaroop VT, Dias L. Orthopedic management of spina bifida. Part I: hip, knee, and rotational deformities. J Child Orthop 2009;3(6):441–9.

43. Chan MC, Khan SA. Ilizarov reconstruction of chronic bilateral calcaneovalgus deformities. Chin J Traumatol 2019;22(4):202–6.

44. Vincent KA. Tarsal coalition and painful flatfoot. J Am Acad Orthop Surg 1998; 6(5):274–81.

45. Lamb D. The ball and socket joint: a congenital abnormality. J Bone Joint Surg Br 1958;40-B(2):240–3.

46. Cho BK, Park KJ, Choi SM, et al. Ankle fusion combined with calcaneal sliding osteotomy for severe arthritis ball and socket ankle deformity. Foot Ankle Int 2016;37(12):1310–6.

47. Ellington JK, Myerson MS. Surgical correction of the ball and socket ankle joint in the adult associated with a talonavicular tarsal coalition. Foot Ankle Int 2013; 34(10):1381–8.

48. Solan MC, Kohls-Gatzoulis J, Stephens MM. Idiopathic toe walking and contractures of the triceps surae. Foot Ankle Clin 2010;15(2):297–307.

49. Knupp M, Schuh R, Stufkens SA, et al. Subtalar and talonavicular arthrodesis through a single medial approach for the correction of severe planovalgus deformity. J Bone Joint Surg Br 2009;91(5):612–5.

50. Jeng CL, Vora AM, Myerson MS. The medial approach to triple arthrodesis. Indications and technique for management of rigid valgus deformities in high-risk patients. Foot Ankle Clin 2005;10(3):515–21, vi–vii.

51. Jeng CL, Tankson CJ, Myerson MS. The single medial approach to triple arthrodesis: a cadaver study. Foot Ankle Int 2006;27(12):1122–5.
52. Jackson WF, Tryfonidis M, Cooke PH, et al. Arthrodesis of the hindfoot for valgus deformity. An entirely medial approach. J Bone Joint Surg Br 2007;89(7):925–7.
53. Saville P, Longman CF, Srinivasan SC, et al. Medial approach for hindfoot arthrodesis with a valgus deformity. Foot Ankle Int 2011;32(8):818–21.
54. Philippot R, Wegrzyn J, Besse JL. Arthrodesis of the subtalar and talonavicular joints through a medial surgical approach: a series of 15 cases. Arch Orthop Trauma Surg 2010;130(5):599–603.
55. Brilhault J. Single medial approach to modified double arthrodesis in rigid flatfoot with lateral deficient skin. Foot Ankle Int 2009;30(1):21–6.
56. Catanzariti AR, Adeleke AT. Double arthrodesis through a medial approach for end-stage adult-acquired flatfoot. Clin Podiatr Med Surg 2014;31(3):435–44.
57. Widnall J, Mason L, Molloy A. Medial approach to the subtalar joint. Foot Ankle Clin 2018;23(3):451–60.
58. Galli MM, Scott RT, Bussewitz B, et al. Structures at risk with medial double hindfoot fusion: a cadaveric study. J Foot Ankle Surg 2014;53(5):598–600.
59. Phisitkul P, Haugsdal J, Vaseenon T, et al. Vascular disruption of the talus: comparison of two approaches for triple arthrodesis. Foot Ankle Int 2013;34(4):568–74.
60. Weinraub GM, Schuberth JM, Lee M, et al. Isolated medial incisional approach to subtalar and talonavicular arthrodesis. J Foot Ankle Surg 2010;49(4):326–30.
61. DeVries JG, Scharer B. Hindfoot deformity corrected with double versus triple arthrodesis: radiographic comparison. J Foot Ankle Surg 2015;54(3):424–7.

Correction of the Neglected Clubfoot in the Adolescent and Adult Patient

Nicholas Peterson, MBChB (Hons), FRCS (Orth)[a,b],*,
Christopher Prior, MBChB, FRCS (Orth)[b]

KEYWORDS

- Clubfoot • Neglected • Relapsed • Equinovarus • Talipes • Salvage • Ilizarov
- Open release

KEY POINTS

- Clubfoot is a 4-dimensional condition: time influences both the severity of the deformity and the success of treatment.
- The Ponseti method was designed for infants; however, it also should be considered alongside alternative strategies for the management of neglected clubfoot.
- Older patients and those with rigid deformities should be considered carefully for gradual correction with external devices, soft tissue release, osteotomies, or fusion procedures.
- A combination of treatments may help to reduce complications and achieve the desired outcome of a pain-free, plantigrade foot.

INTRODUCTION

The clubfoot deformity consists of varying degrees of hindfoot varus and equinus with cavus, forefoot adduction, and internal rotation.[1–3] Idiopathic clubfoot, or congenital talipes equinovarus (CTEV), occurs in 1/1000 to 2/1000 live births.[4–6] In high-income countries, the condition is identified prenatally by ultrasound and followed with early neonatal treatment.[7] There is a multifactorial etiology with genetic, environmental, vascular, and embryologic factors likely.[8] Aside from the idiopathic variety, the clubfoot deformity may be secondary to myelomeningocele, arthrogryposis, hereditary motor and sensory neuropathies, and other neuromuscular disorders.[2]

There are intraosseous and interosseous deformities in clubfoot. The lateral malleolus of the fibula lies posteriorly in relation to the distal tibia; this may be a primary deformity or simply a reflection of the body of the talus lying in external rotation to the tibia.[9]

[a] Royal Liverpool & Broadgreen University Hospital, Liverpool, UK; [b] Alder Hey Children's Hospital, East Prescot Road, Liverpool L14 5AB, UK
* Corresponding author. Alder Hey Children's Hospital, East Prescot Road, Liverpool L14 5AB, UK.
E-mail address: Nicholas.D.Peterson@alderhey.nhs.uk

Foot Ankle Clin N Am 25 (2020) 205–220
https://doi.org/10.1016/j.fcl.2020.02.008
1083-7515/20/Crown Copyright © 2020 Published by Elsevier Inc. All rights reserved.

foot.theclinics.com

The talus is uncovered anteriorly and laterally due to the equinovarus position at the ankle, and the neck is dysplastic and internally rotated relative to the body. The navicular is subluxed medially around the talar head and may abut the medial malleolus. The calcaneum is small, internally rotated, and supinated, with an oblique calcaneocuboid joint that leaves the cuboid medially subluxed. Although the existence of tibial internal rotation[10] and the position of the talar body in the ankle mortise are not agreed on among all investigators,[6,9] magnetic resonance imaging (MRI) studies suggest the talar body is rotated externally and the neck has rotated internally.[9,11]

Clubfoot is a 4-dimensional problem: spatial and temporal. Time changes the nature of the deformity and eventual prognosis. Development of osseous anatomy in a child's foot depends on transmission of force through congruent and anatomically aligned articulations. Untreated, or if treated inadequately, the bones in the clubfoot become ossified while malaligned and exposed to abnormal forces, adding to the abnormal bony anatomy, described previously. This important distinction separates the clubfoot presenting early for management from that presenting late; in the latter, whether untreated or neglected by failed previous treatment, the foot shape may not be improved sufficiently without resort to osteotomy if the remodeling potential of growing bone is lost.[6]

Neglected clubfoot can be defined as cases untreated until after a child begins to walk,[12] although some investigators consider no treatment before age 2 or 3 as qualifying.[4,13] This is seen commonly in low-income countries where health inequalities and the distances of some rural communities from suitable clinics are large.[6,14] The neglected clubfoot worsens over time due to the forces transmitted through the malpositioned foot during ambulation; in extreme cases, the foot faces backward, with the patient walking on the dorsum of the foot. Painful callosities develop on the unsuitable dorsal skin of the foot, which then breaks down and becomes infected. The foot progressively becomes more difficult to shod and to treat.[6]

Recurrence is, despite treatment, common; the underlying cause is seldom removed. Long-term follow-up reveals a recurrence rate requiring surgical intervention of between 30% and 45% in idiopathic CTEV.[15–17] Recurrence rates are higher in patients with secondary clubfoot deformity.[18] Treatment of recurrent or unsuccessfully treated CTEV shares the same principles with treating the neglected clubfoot. In both, secondary changes have occurred after growth that add to the deformity.

ROLE OF THE PONSETI METHOD IN NEGLECTED CLUBFOOT

The Ponseti technique uses the viscoelastic properties of ligaments and tendons in order to bring about the sequential correction of cavus, adduction, varus, and equinus. Foot manipulations held for a few minutes prior to casting allow stress relaxation of the soft tissue structures before an above-knee cast is applied.[19] In idiopathic CTEV, correction of a responsive clubfoot deformity may take 5 to 6 casts and an Achilles tendon release is required in more than 80% of cases to correct the equinus without causing a rocker-bottom deformity.[1] There must follow 3 to 4 months of continuous bracing, with the feet held in abduction and dorsiflexion by boots and bars. Thereafter, boots and bars are continued for nights and naps up to age 4 or 5. Failures and recurrence of the deformity are frequently due to a lack of compliance.[8]

This method of treatment has an initial success rate of more than 90% for idiopathic CTEV.[20] An accurate reproduction of the treatment protocol as well as patient compliance are needed but the Ponseti method is cheap and effective.[21] Success is lower in cases of clubfoot secondary to other pathology and management usually follows a more complicated course in these patients.[18]

Ponseti's original publication described treatment of patients up the age of 6 months, with an average age of 1 month.[1] Successful outcomes in older children have been reported[21–24] with 1 article demonstrating bony remodeling (through MRI) in a child of 7 years with correction maintained after 2.5 years' follow-up.[25] This suggests that if the technique is tolerated by patients and families, it is an excellent option due to the low costs and low risks. It can be attempted in older children although the upper age limit for effectiveness is not known.[4]

Modifications in the Ponseti method for neglected clubfoot have included greater numbers of serial treatments, longer periods of casting, longer manipulations, and the use of ankle-foot orthoses (AFOs) rather than boots and bars.[12,21] Encouraging results have been demonstrated for patients up to 12 years of age with these techniques, although results are better for younger patients and for deformities of the forefoot rather than hindfoot.[21] Nunn and colleagues[14] have developed the plantaris, adduction, varus, equinus, and rotation (PAVER) score in order to predict which children with neglected clubfoot will respond to Ponseti treatment. They combine the Diméglio classification measurements with a multiplier for the age of the patient in order to give a score out of 30.[26] Only 1 child in their cohort with a score of more than 18/30 was fully corrected by closed means compared with a high success rate with lower scores.[14]

An assessment of benefit from partially successful serial cast treatment needs to be balanced against the need for further surgery in order to achieve fully the aims of clubfoot treatment. It is almost certainly a decision that has to be individualized.[4,6,12,14,24]

GRADUAL CORRECTION BY EXTERNAL FIXATION

Nunn's PAVER score may identify those cases where serial casting is likely to not be successful. In rigid deformities, particularly in older children[2,14] and in those where previous open surgery has been performed and has led to extensive scarring, the Ilizarov method offers hope of correction but even this method may have to be combined with minimal open releases, osteotomies, and selected joint arthrodesis after correction (usually at the subtalar or midfoot).

If there is expertise and infrastructure available, and the patient and family are suitable for this method of treatment, gradual correction by an external fixator can offer hope of significant improvement. The principles of distraction histogenesis have been demonstrated using a variety of fixators,[27] although the Ilizarov device has versatility to correct all components of the deformity simultaneously.

The Ilizarov circular external fixator has been used for treating nonidiopathic CTEV and chronic or complex relapses[28–30] of the condition. It can be used with limited surgical releases of soft tissues as a minimally invasive technique that reduces scarring and thus maintains the plasticity of the tissues.[2] With the Ilizarov method, the deformities of clubfoot are treated simultaneously rather than sequentially with the speed of correction titrated to patient tolerance. The method requires experience with the application and postoperative management of circular external fixation for deformity correction in order to avoid complications such as joint subluxation, iatrogenic physeal separation, or an incomplete correction.

Although surgeons may have individual preferences when using the Ilizarov technique for neglected or resistant CTEV, the authors describe the steps they use. The indications are severe, stiff deformities of the foot that have been treated before (either by the sequence of procedures comprising the Ponseti method or by classic open surgical releases) or even in neglected CTEV (although this is seen uncommonly in the United Kingdom).

Preparation

Anaesthesia should be without continuous muscle paralysis in order to enable intraoperative monitoring for nerve injury when passing wires. After standard preparation and drape, a sterile thigh tourniquet is applied.

Stage 1: Plantar Fascia Release

With the limb exsanguinated and tourniquet inflated, the plantar fascia is identified using a semicircular incision centered around the calcaneal tuberosity on the plantar aspect of the foot (**Fig. 1**). The incision is distal to the point of heel contact. Sharp dissection through skin and fat is made until the fibers of the plantar fascia are visualized directly. The plantar fascia and intrinsic muscles are divided sharply to the plantar surface of the calcaneum just distal to the tuberosity with care to avoid injury to the lateral and medial plantar nerves (located more distal to the area of dissection). Skin closure is followed with a crepe bandage before releasing the tourniquet.

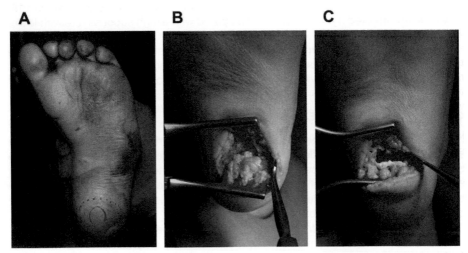

A   **B**   **C**

Fig. 1. (*A*) Incision for plantar fascia release with the palpable calcaneal tuberosity marked and the incision curved approximately 15 mm to 20 mm anteriorly. (*B*) The incision is deepened to fascia and (*C*) the fascia and origin of intrinsic muscles from the tuberosity divided.

Stage 2: Circular External Fixator Application

The circular external fixator has 3 main assemblies: tibial, hindfoot, and forefoot. These are joined by a series of strategically placed hinges and motor units. The tibial segment comprises a 2-ring block, with the distal end being approximately 12-cm proximal to the ankle joint (approximately a handbreadth) (**Fig. 2**). Wires are passed in safe corridors, with the ankle, foot, and toes moved into a position to stretch the muscles of the compartment before the wire is passed through. Sudden contraction or a muscle twitch suggests nerve proximity to the wire; this should prompt a reinsertion of the wire at a different level or position. Small incisions are needed to allow passage of olives, if such wires are used. Dressings and pressure are applied to the pin sites to minimize hematoma formation during the procedure.

An appropriate ring size with 2 fingerbreadths of clearance around the limb is selected and the tibial assembly completed by attaching and tensioning the wires. The wires are tensioned to 110 kg using a tensioning device.

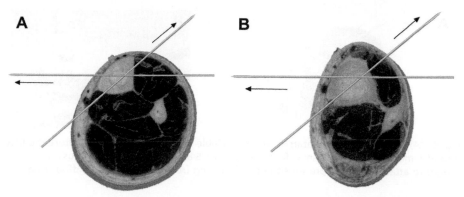

Fig. 2. Safe corridors for coronal plane and medial face wire insertion in the (*A*) middle tibia and (*B*) distal tibia.

Stage 3: Hindfoot Segment

The safe corridors in the hindfoot differ. The bandages around the heel are removed and the posterior tibial artery is palpated and marked out. This can be difficult due to the varus hindfoot position, in which case ultrasound Doppler can be used to mark the artery. The first olive wire is passed with the entry just posterior to the posterior tibial artery and angled anteromedial to posterolateral (**Fig. 3**). A second olive wire is passed from the lateral side from anterolateral to posteromedial, approximately 1-cm posterior and inferior to the tip of the lateral malleolus—a useful tip is to judge the inclination of this wire by viewing the foot from the plantar aspect with the surgeon standing at the foot of the table and holding the wires in position while an assistant controls the wire driver. The inclination can be altered such that a good crossing angle and central location in the calcaneum is achieved.

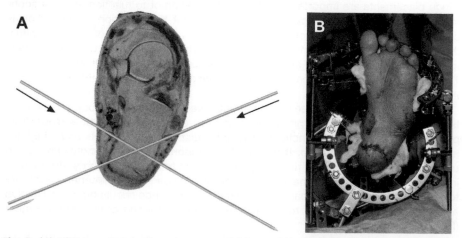

Fig. 3. (*A*) Oblique wires in the calcaneum which provide the hold onto the hindfoot. (*B*) Positioning the 5/8 ring to enable capture of the wires and allow for adequate clearance around the foot. ([A] *Modified from* Nayagam S. Safe corridors in external fixation: the lower leg (tibia, fibula, hindfoot and forefoot). *Strategies Trauma Limb Reconstr.* 2007;2(2-3):105–110.)

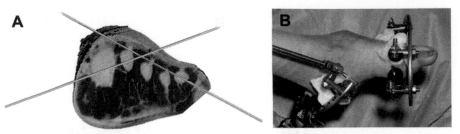

Fig. 4. (*A*) The fixation of metatarsals can be variable but it is important to capture the first and fifth metatarsals. (*B*) In a small foot, moving the 5/8 ring more distally and using posts or hinges to attach the wires prevents the forefoot ring from abutting the hindfoot ring.

These wires are attached to a 5/8 ring, which is set to approximate the inclination of hindfoot—usually varus and equinus. In severe equinus or osteopenic bone, an additional wire or a single half-pin in the long axis of the calcaneus improves fixation strength.

Stage 4: Forefoot Segment

The heads of the metatarsals are palpated and marked on the skin to serve as a visual guide. The medial olive wire is passed through the first metatarsal and aimed to pass through the distal third of the second and third metatarsals, directed from inferomedial to dorsolateral, and avoiding the distal physes of the metatarsals. Again, an assistant operates the wire driver while the surgeon palpates each metatarsal with thumb and finger to stabilize the bone during wire passage. A second wire is passed from the neck of the fifth metatarsal toward the first metatarsal from inferolateral to dorsomedial. The wires are attached to a 5/8 ring, which is positioned orthogonal to the long axis of the metatarsals (**Fig. 4**).

Stage 5: Connecting the Tibial and Hindfoot Segments

Hinge placements are important for the Ilizarov construct to function as a semiconstrained correcting device; by this, it is meant that the direction of correction is controlled partly by the location of hinges and partly by the shape of the joints within the foot. Hindfoot correction involves positioning 3 hinges. The first 2 are either universal or biplanar hinges located at the level of the tips of the lateral and medial malleoli. This transmalleolar axis replicates the axis of the ankle joint. These are connected to the tibial ring block (**Fig. 5**).

Next, a motor unit to increase the distance between the tibial ring block and the posterior aspect of the hindfoot ring is needed—this drives correction of equinus. This posterior motor unit has 2 functions: it enables distraction but it acts as a hinge for hindfoot varus correction too. It is, therefore, important that this motor and hinge unit is placed on the hindfoot ring in a position close to the subtalar axis. An approximate location to this axis is the inferior posterolateral part of the calcaneal tuberosity to the superior anteromedial part of the talar neck. The hinge should be placed on this axis and the posterior motor rod connected to the distal ring of the tibial segment (**Fig. 6**).

Stage 6: Connecting the Hindfoot and Forefoot Segments

Two motor units connect the hindfoot to forefoot segments to correct forefoot adduction and cavus. Connections on the medial and lateral sides are via hinges on the end of posts dropped plantarward on either side of the hindfoot ring. The rods are parallel

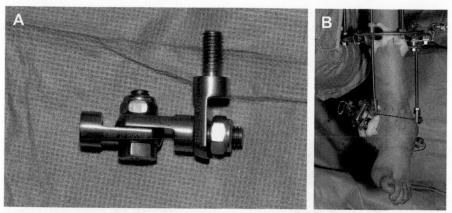

Fig. 5. (*A*) A biplanar hinge is constructed from 2 male posts and 1 female post held with threaded nuts with a nylon insert. If this is attached to the ring with another nut with nylon insert, then it functions as a triplanar or universal hinge. (*B*) Two biplanar hinges are placed on the calcaneal ring directly opposite the tips of the malleoli to simulate the axis of the ankle joint (*arrow*).

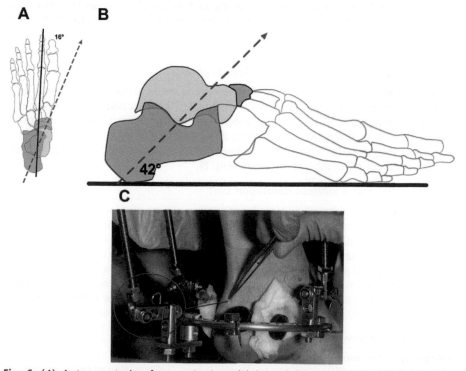

Fig. 6. (*A*) Anteroposterior foot projection. (*B*) lateral foot projection. Identifying the approximate position of the axis of the subtalar joint in the axial and sagittal planes. Approximately, it lies between the posterolateral corner of the calcaneum to the anteromedial part of the neck of the talus. (*C*) The posterior hinge (biplanar) is placed at the level distal to the posterior facet (shown by forceps) of the subtalar joint and rotated to approximate the axis.

to the sole of the foot to facilitate distraction along this direction. These rods terminate on the forefoot ring via universal (triplanar) hinges (**Fig. 7**).

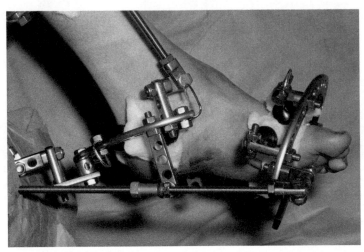

Fig. 7. Rods, which lie parallel to the sole of the foot (horizontally), drive the metatarsal ring from the calcaneal ring. Different rates of lengthening between medial and lateral rods can correct forefoot adduction.

Stage 7: Connecting the Tibial and Forefoot Segments

The forefoot segment is connected via 2 anterior rods linked to the tibial assembly by a T construct comprising a twisted and long plate bolted together and at the anterior end are two 4-hole posts (male and female) linked together via washers. This arrangement enables correction of plantaris (forefoot equinus) and forefoot supination. The motor units are outrigged in this manner so that their direction of pull is tangential to a circle around the center of rotation at the ankle (**Fig. 8**).

Stage 8: Addition of a midfoot derotation unit

Addition of a midfoot derotation unit is for producing a correction of internal rotation of the forefoot, which is a deformity occurring at the midfoot joints. Because the T construct is attached to the tibial ring at a position overlying the center of the head of the talus (or anyway along the bisector line; see **Fig. 11**), when a motor rod unit is linked to the medial side of the T construct via a hinge it allows a push mechanism for derotation (shown in **Fig. 9**). With rotation of the T construct around an axis over the center of the head of the talus, the forefoot is able to derotate from internal to external. This usually is the final stage of correction.

Stage 9: Postoperative Correction

Preliminary ankle joint arthrodiatasis
With pain management and pin site care established,[31] distraction of the ankle joint is started by lengthening all 5 motor units that link the tibial segment to the hindfoot and forefoot. This is at a rate of one-fourth turn, 4 times daily (total 1 mm per day). Ankle joint distraction avoids iatrogenic compression of the articular cartilage during correction and anterior talar body subluxation during equinus correction. After ankle distraction (usually 1 week), lateral radiographs of the ankle confirm the widened joint space

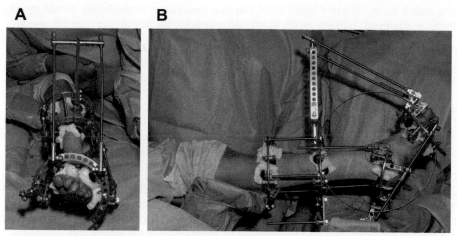

Fig. 8. (*A*) The forefoot segment (metatarsal ring) is connected to the tibial segment via 2 long anterior rods and a T assembly constructed of a twisted plate, long straight plate, and male and female posts coupled together. (*B*) Lateral view of connection between the tibial and forefoot segments. Shortening of the long anterior rods pulls the forefoot from equinus at a tangent to an arc which subtends the center of rotation of the ankle.

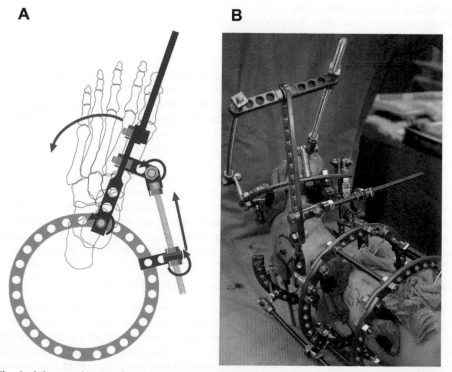

Fig. 9. (*A*) A mechanism for derotating the forefoot around the head of the talus. (*B*) Here the attachment of the T construct to the tibial ring is on the bisector line of the deformity of which the CORA is located around the center of the head of the talus (refer to **Fig. 11**).

and check for inadvertent distal tibial physeal separation in skeletally immature patients; if observed, percutaneous Kirschner wires across the physis may be needed.

Correcting hindfoot equinus and forefoot equinus (plantaris)
By lengthening the posterior rod that links the tibial to hindfoot assembly and the 2 medial and lateral horizontal rods that link hindfoot to forefoot segments, while simultaneously shortening the 2 long anterior rods that sit astride the T construct, the deformities, hindfoot equinus and forefoot equinus (plantaris), are corrected gradually. The usual rates are 1 mm per day of lengthening on the posterior and horizontal rods and 3 mm per day of shortening of the anterior long rods. The changes to length of the rods are done in fractions several times daily in keeping with Ilizarov principles.

Correcting forefoot adduction
Once plantaris is corrected, relative lengthening of the medial horizontal rod over that of the lateral one leads to correction of the forefoot adduction. If radiographs reveal excessive joint diatasis in the joints of the midfoot and forefoot, then lengthening of the medial horizontal rod can be coupled to shortening of the lateral rod.

Correcting hindfoot varus
On correction of hindfoot equinus, a relative lengthening of the medial posterior rod (linked to the medial hinge that is positioned over the tip of the medial malleolus) over that of the lateral posterior rod allows rotation of the calcaneum around the hinge construct positioned posteriorly, in line with the axis of the subtalar joint.

Correcting forefoot supination
When plantaris is corrected, a greater amount of shortening of the lateral long anterior rod relative to the medial corrects supination.

Correcting forefoot internal rotation
The final phase is the correction of internal rotation of the forefoot by lengthening the outrigged motor unit on the medial side of the T construct.

In severe deformities, it may take 3 months for gradual correction to complete to a position of over-correction (this is a desired objective) and another 6 weeks to maintain this posture of the foot and ankle. At times, an adjustment of the foot and fixator under anesthesia as a day case is needed (often in midcorrection phase) to facilitate further progress when there appears to be a stall in the changes in the position of the foot.

A molded cast is applied at time of frame removal and the foot held in an over-corrected position in the cast for 6 weeks. Thereafter, mobilization of the foot and ankle by physiotherapy commences together with a regime of splintage in a neutral AFO splint for daytime use; at night, the authors use an AFO molded with some over-correction incorporated. The authors maintain daytime splintage for 6 months and whereas night-time splintage continues until after the pubertal growth spurt.

OPEN SURGERY UTILIZING SOFT TISSUE RELEASES AND OSTEOTOMIES

The PAVER score[14] may indicate when a clubfoot requires operative intervention. Penny[6] described a simple classification system for neglected clubfoot with 3 categories: moderately flexible, moderately stiff, and rigid. These descriptors can be applied to the deformities of the hindfoot and midfoot. Open surgery may be indicated for those moderately stiff deformities where the Ponseti method may not be successful on its own or for those children in whom the Ilizarov method of treatment may be unsuited.

Extensive open surgery has fallen out of favor with the advent and popularity of the Ponseti method. Despite the association with scarring and risks of injury to neurovascular structures, however, it is not without merit. It can be used as part of a staged approach, which begins with either serial casting or gradual correction by external fixation, with the aim of reducing the magnitude and resistance of the contractures and deformity prior to open surgery, when less extensive releases then are required.[24,32]

While planning open releases, the following points need to be considered:

1. Age: older children and adolescents are likely to have more established contractures resistant to simple soft tissue releases as well as changes to bone shape. Osteotomy is more likely to be needed.
2. Flexibility: the more rigid deformities may require preoperative serial casting to deliver some degree of correction first. Osteotomy also is more likely.
3. Anatomy: the contractures leading to the components of a CTEV deformity lie in the ankle and subtalar joints, midfoot joints, and plantar fascia. Access to these structures must be part of the surgical plan.
4. Muscle imbalance: loss of muscle control across the ankle and subtalar joints may be partially responsible for the deformity in the first instance. A clinical examination performed in the months after deformity correction is completed may indicate where the imbalance lies. Appropriate and timely tendon transfers can prevent early relapse.

The approach the authors advocate is based on that described previously by Carroll,[33] which uses 2 incisions. Both incisions and the deep dissection that follow can be done in the prone position or in the lateral position first (for the posterolateral incision) and then supine (for the medial incision).

Through the Posterolateral Incision

The skin incision lies between the lateral edge of the Achilles tendon and the fibula. The sural nerve and the short saphenous vein are dissected free and retracted. A Z-lengthening is carried out on the Achilles tendon with the distal transverse limb of the Z cut medially. For neglected clubfeet, a release of the ankle and subtalar joints should follow.

The interval between the flexor hallucis longus and peroneus brevis is developed to enable the ability to retract flexor hallucis longus and the posterior tibial neurovascular bundle medially and expose the posterior aspects of the ankle and subtalar joint.

Arthrotomies of the ankle and subtalar joints are carried out. Three deep ligaments that require division are

1. The posterior tibiofibular ligament, which allows the body of the talus to rotate into the ankle mortise by allowing the fibula to descend and rotate
2. The posterior talofibular ligament, which also restrains movement of the fibula during attempted dorsiflexion of the ankle
3. The calcaneofibular ligament, which is visualized by lifting the peroneal tendons. This key structure, when contracted, prevents rotation of the calcaneum from varus into valgus. A release is always needed.

When the releases are completed, the heel is then rotated into valgus by abducting the forefoot (as in a Ponseti manoeuvre) before dorsiflexion is attempted. Often, plantigrade or better is achievable at this point (**Fig. 10**).

Through the Medial Incision

The medial skin incision is based around 3 palpable landmarks: the base of the first metatarsal, the medial malleolus, and calcaneal tuberosity. The authors prefer a

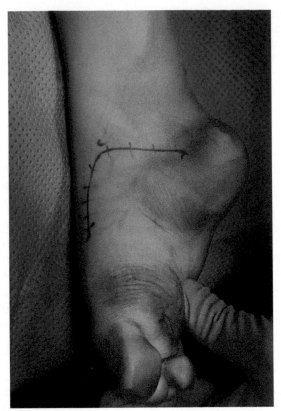

Fig. 10. Surface anatomy for the curvilinear incision to the medial side of the foot marked on a case of recurrent CTEV after failed Ponseti treatment.

curvilinear incision over that described by Carroll[33] because this avoids scar contraction which can contribute to recurrence.

The flap is elevated and turned plantarward. Tibialis posterior tendon and abductor hallucis are important landmarks. The former leads to the talonavicular joint and the latter bridges over the posterior tibial neurovascular bundle. Tibialis posterior is identified proximally and followed distally. Sharp reflection of the abductor hallucis in a plantar direction gives better access to the medial aspect of the foot. The posterior tibial neurovascular bundle is identified and protected. Tibialis posterior tendon is Z-lengthened and the capsule of the talonavicular joint is circumferentially incised. The plantar half of tibialis posterior is traced via its plantar expansion into the sole of the foot. Sharp division of this expansion exposes the master knot of Henry. Further deep dissection in this plane toward the lateral side reaches the medial capsule of the calcaneocuboid joint, which also is incised.

At the posterior end of the incision, posterior to the lateral plantar nerve and vessels (these can be taken forward with a blunt retractor), the plane between the fat of the heel pad and plantar fascia is identified. Sharp division of the plantar fascia is then performed.

In neglected clubfeet, restoration of a straight lateral border to the foot (and adequate correction of forefoot adduction and internal rotation) can be achieved only by a lateral column shortening through the calcaneum. The correct location of the closing wedge that allows for external rotation of the forefoot around the talonavicular joint is between the anterior and middle facets of the subtalar joint (**Fig. 11**). This wedge can be removed through a lateral longitudinal incision starting at the anterior process of the calcaneum and extended posteriorly. Extensor digitorum brevis is elevated anteriorly and the peroneal tendons retracted plantarward. An osteotome then is directed to just anterior to the sustentaculum tali (middle facet of subtalar joint) to create one side of the wedge to be removed.

Fixation of the closing wedge osteotomy may be achieved with a lateral plate or Kirschner wires in the younger patient.

SALVAGE PROCEDURES

Salvage procedures comprise a variety of osteotomies through the calcaneum (lateral translation and Dwyer lateral closing wedge), arthrodesis of the midfoot or hindfoot (usually the triple arthrodesis), and even osteotomy-distraction with an Ilizarov fixator (often via a V-osteotomy or U-osteotomy).[34] These procedures are unlikely to be needed in a neglected clubfoot, even one that is recurrent after treatment, because the absence of dense scarring lends itself to successful treatment by one of the methods described previously: the Ponseti technique, open releases with osteotomy

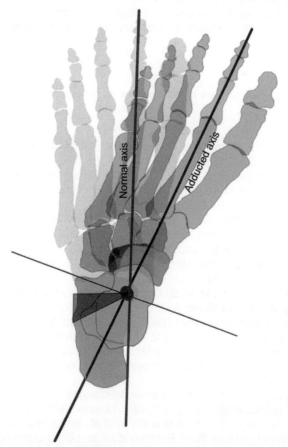

Fig. 11. Lateral closing wedge positioned with the apex between the anterior and middle facets of the subtalar joint of the calcaneum.

or closed treatment and gradual correction with the Ilizarov fixator. Only in cases of dense scarring or severe resistant clubfoot is resort to these salvage procedures needed.

SUMMARY

Neglected, recurrent, or relapsed clubfoot is a major treatment challenge due to the complex 4-dimensional nature of the problem. The congenital basis of the condition prevents complete restoration of normal anatomy; therefore, the focus is on achieving pain-free function rather than radiographic or cosmetic perfection. Less invasive methods producing incremental gradual improvements in foot shape and joint alignment, such as the Ponseti and Ilizarov, are preferred. Open surgery with or without osteotomy then can be limited to those moderately stiff clubfeet in patients unsuited to treatment using the Ilizarov method or unlikely to be corrected completely by the Ponseti technique.

ACKNOWLEDGEMENTS

The authors would like to acknowledge and thank Mr Selvadurai Nayagam for his expert advice and guidance throughout the preparation of this article. We are indebted to him for sharing the insights and understanding he has gained from a career treating patients with clubfoot. We particularly thank him for the illustrations he has provided for this work.

DISCLOSURE

N. Peterson and C. Prior declare no financial or commercial conflicts of interest.

REFERENCES

1. Ponseti I, Smoley E. Congenital club foot: the results of treatment. J Bone Joint Surg Am 1963;45(2):83.
2. Malizos KN, Gougoulias NE, Dailiana ZH, et al. Relapsed clubfoot correction with soft-tissue release and selective application of Ilizarov technique. Strategies Trauma Limb Reconstr 2008;3(3):109–17.
3. Herold HZ, Torok G. Surgical correction of neglected club foot in the older child and adult. J Bone Joint Surg Am 1973;55(7):1385–95.
4. Digge V, Desai J, Das S. Expanded age indication for ponseti method for correction of congenital idiopathic talipes equinovarus: a systematic review. J Foot Ankle Surg 2018;57(1):155–8.
5. Wang H, Barisic I, Loane M, et al. Congenital clubfoot in Europe: a population-based study. Am J Med Genet A 2019;179(4):595–601.
6. Penny J. The neglected clubfoot. Tech Orthop 2005;20(2):14.
7. Faldini C, Fenga D, Sanzarello I, et al. Prenatal diagnosis of clubfoot: a review of current available methodology. Folia Med (Plovdiv) 2017;59(3):247–53.
8. Herring JA. Tachdjian's pediatric orthopedics. 5th editon. Philadelphia: Elsevier Saunders; 2014.
9. Herzenberg JE, Carroll NC, Christofersen MR, et al. Clubfoot analysis with three-dimensional computer modeling. J Pediatr Orthop 1988;8(3):257–62.
10. Windisch G, Anderhuber F, Haldi-Brändle V, et al. Anatomical study for an update comprehension of clubfoot. Part I: Bones and joints. J Child Orthop 2007;1(1):69–77.
11. Song HR, Carroll NC, Neyt J, et al. Clubfoot analysis with three-dimensional foot models. J Pediatr Orthop B 1999;8(1):5–11.

12. Mehtani A, Prakash J, Vijay V, et al. Modified Ponseti technique for management of neglected clubfeet. J Pediatr Orthop B 2018;27(1):61–6.

13. Sengupta A. The management of congenital talipes equinovarus in developing countries. Int Orthop 1987;11(3):183–7.

14. Nunn TR, Etsub M, Tilahun T, et al. Development and validation of a delayed presenting clubfoot score to predict the response to Ponseti casting for children aged 2-10. Strateg Trauma Limb Reconstr 2018;13(3):171–7.

15. Cooper DM, Dietz FR. Treatment of idiopathic clubfoot. A thirty-year follow-up note. J Bone Joint Surg Am 1995;77(10):1477–89.

16. Bor N, Coplan JA, Herzenberg JE. Ponseti treatment for idiopathic clubfoot: minimum 5-year followup. Clin Orthop Relat Res 2009;467(5):1263–70.

17. Gelfer Y, Wientroub S, Hughes K, et al. Congenital talipes equinovarus: a systematic review of relapse as a primary outcome of the Ponseti method. Bone Joint J 2019;101-B(6):639–45.

18. Matar HE, Makki D, Garg NK. Treatment of syndrome-associated congenital talipes equinovarus using the Ponseti method: 4-12 years of follow-up. J Pediatr Orthop B 2018;27(1):56–60.

19. Cummings RJ, Davidson RS, Armstrong PF, et al. Congenital clubfoot. J Bone Joint Surg Am 2002;84(2):290–308.

20. Morcuende JA, Dolan LA, Dietz FR, et al. Radical reduction in the rate of extensive corrective surgery for clubfoot using the Ponseti method. Pediatrics 2004; 113(2):376–80.

21. Lourenço AF, Morcuende JA. Correction of neglected idiopathic club foot by the Ponseti method. J Bone Joint Surg Br 2007;89(3):378–81.

22. Spiegel DA, Shrestha OP, Sitoula P, et al. Ponseti method for untreated idiopathic clubfeet in Nepalese patients from 1 to 6 years of age. Clin Orthop Relat Res 2009;467(5):1164–70.

23. Khan SA, Kumar A. Ponseti's manipulation in neglected clubfoot in children more than 7 years of age: a prospective evaluation of 25 feet with long-term follow-up. J Pediatr Orthop B 2010;19(5):385–9.

24. Ayana B, Klungsoyr P. Good results after Ponsetitreatment for neglected congenital clubfoot in Ethiopia. Acta Orthop 2014;85(6):5.

25. Nogueira MP, Amaral DT. How much remodeling is possible in a clubfoot treatment? Magnetic resonance imaging study in a 7-year-old child. J Limb Lengthen Reconstr 2018;4:49–54.

26. Diméglio A, Bensahel H, Souchet P, et al. Classification of clubfoot. J Pediatr Orthop B 1995;4(2):129–36.

27. Singh A. Evaluation of neglected idiopathic ctev managed by ligamentotaxis using jess: a long-term followup. Adv Orthop 2011;2011:218489.

28. Ferreira RC, Costo MT, Frizzo GG, et al. Correction of neglected clubfoot using the Ilizarov external fixator. Foot Ankle Int 2006;27(4):266–73.

29. El Barbary H, Abdel Ghani H, Hegazy M. Correction of relapsed or neglected clubfoot using a simple Ilizarov frame. Int Orthop 2004;28(3):183–6.

30. Grill F, Franke J. The Ilizarov distractor for the correction of relapsed or neglected clubfoot. J Bone Joint Surg Br 1987;69-B(4):593–7.

31. Davies R, Holt N, Nayagam S. The care of pin sites with external fixation. J Bone Joint Surg Br 2005;87(5):716–9.

32. Emara K, El Moatasem eH, El Shazly O. Correction of complex equino cavo varus foot deformity in skeletally mature patients by Ilizarov external fixation versus staged external-internal fixation. Foot Ankle Surg 2011;17(4):287–93.
33. Carroll NC. Pathoanatomy and surgical treatment of the resistant clubfoot. Instr Course Lect 1988;37:93–106.
34. Shalaby H, Hefny H. Correction of complex foot deformities using the V-osteotomy and the Ilizarov technique. Strateg Trauma Limb Reconstr 2007; 2(1):21–30.

Reconstruction of Severe Ankle and Pilon Fracture Malunions

Ben Fischer, FRCS (Tr&Orth)[a,b,*],
Lyndon William Mason, MB BCh, MRCS (eng), FRCS (Tr&Orth), FRCS (Glasg)[a,c]

KEYWORDS

- Pilon fracture • Ankle fracture • Malunion • Reconstruction • Osteotomy

KEY POINTS

- Malunion of ankle and pilon fractures has significant detrimental effect on function and development of post-trauma osteoarthritis.
- Pilon and ankle malunions can occur at one of three levels: mechanical axis deformity in the metaphysis/supramalleolar region, periarticular zone (including joint incongruity), or in the hindfoot.
- Common osteotomies to correct malalignment include supramalleolar wedge osteotomy, supramalleolar dome osteotomy, fibular osteotomy, plafond-plasty, periarticular osteotomy, and calcaneal osteotomy.

INTRODUCTION

High-energy fractures of the distal tibia, the tibial plafond, and involving the ankle mortise are uncommon injuries, occurring in approximately 7% of tibia fractures.[1] Most commonly, these fractures relate to a mechanism of large energy transfer where an axial force is applied to the distal tibia, with an additional rotational moment around the ankle mortise.[2,3] The vector, in which the axial load is transmitted across the plafond, the position of the foot at the time of the injury, and pretensioning of the Achilles tendon relates to the severity and orientation of the fracture fragments. Energy dissipates across the distal tibia causing fracture not only of the articular surface but also the metaphysis above and occasionally the foot below.[4] Several methods of surgical treatment have been proposed, with the aim of treatment being to restore the articular

[a] Trauma and Orthopaedic Department, Aintree University Hospital, Lower Lane, Liverpool L9 7AL, UK; [b] Mersey Ortho-plastic Group, Liverpool Limb Reconstruction Service; [c] University of Liverpool, Liverpool, UK
* Corresponding author. Trauma and Orthopaedic Department, Aintree University Hospital, Lower Lane, Liverpool L9 7AL, UK.
E-mail address: benjamin.fischer@aintree.nhs.uk
Twitter: drlyndonmason (L.W.M.)

Foot Ankle Clin N Am 25 (2020) 221–237
https://doi.org/10.1016/j.fcl.2020.02.007

congruency and maintain alignment of the weight-bearing axis.[1,2,5] Success depends on considered decision-making, planning, and accurate surgical technique. Although these injuries represent a small fraction of the fracture workload, they do require an inversely proportional, inordinate degree of surgical effort to minimize complications and maximize results.

The energy dissipated within the bony anatomy is transferred to the local soft tissue envelope, manifest in an indirect fashion, shearing of the tissue layers, or by direct injury; in-to-out, or out-to-in wounds.[6] The soft tissue envelope insult alone relates to poor outcomes, and may dictate primary surgical choice and enforce the acceptance of poor orthogonal correction in the initial treatment. Fractures associated with osteoporosis present their own challenges, often with comorbidity, poor premorbid soft tissues; high-energy injury patterns relating to low-energy mechanism and preexisting joint pathology. Dujardin and colleagues[2] in their review of surgical interventions for pilon fractures reported imperfect articular reduction to occur in 0% to 25% and nonarticular malunion of 0% to 9.5%. Higher rates of malunion have been reported in the use of bridging external fixation without articular fixation, and the use of lateral internal plate fixation.[2]

Ankle fractures in contrast, are one of the most common injuries presenting to an orthopedic trauma department. The injuries are often underestimated, with a reported malreduction rate reported to be 44%.[7,8] Whitehouse and colleagues[7] reported that there was a culture of "it's just an ankle" in the surgical treatment, leading to poor reduction and subsequent malunion. Roberts and colleagues[8] reported a significant reduction in patient function in individuals malreduced at time of surgery once again concluding that the underappreciation of the injury was critical in the poor outcome.

PRESENTATION AND PLANNING

Malunions of the distal tibia and ankle can occur exclusively intra-articular, exclusively extra-articular, or a combination of both. The tibia, fibular, and ligamentous restraints can each be affected to varying degrees. Patients present with pain, loss of function, and/or deformity. On assessment, it is essential to assess the patient as a whole, but particularly focusing on their problematic limb. The cutaneous stigmata of the primary injury, and previous surgical scars should be documented. Leg length discrepancy and foot orientation should be reviewed. Assessment of heel position, ankle motion, subtalar motion, and general gait can give indicators to underlying pathology. The malleolar position should be assessed in comparison with the contralateral side.

On further investigation, adequate long leg alignment views should be obtained, from hip to heel with both patellae pointing anteriorly. Weight-bearing radiographs of the ankle and hindfoot alignment views (eg, Saltzman view)[9] allow identification of level of true deformity and compensatory deformity (**Fig. 1**). Computed tomography (CT) is a vital means of assessing degree of union, anatomy of malunion, and intra-articular pathology. Three-dimensional (3D) rendered CT images are useful, allowing a greater perception and understanding of the deformity; however, this image is static and may hide deformity dependent of weight-bearing position (**Fig. 2**). The use of weight-bearing CT has further enhanced the diagnostic accuracy of hind foot alignment assessment, introducing the parameter, foot ankle offset. Lintz and colleagues[10] found that in normal cases, the mean value for foot ankle offset was 2.3% ± 2.9%, whereas in varus and valgus cases, the mean was −11.6% ± 6.9% and 11.4% ± 5.7%, Unfortunately, this assessment is not widely available.

Other recent technological advances have meant that 3D print reconstructions of the deformity can be produced (**Fig. 3**).[11] This is particularly beneficial for malunion

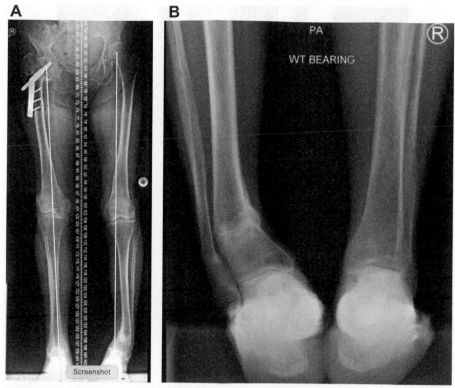

Fig. 1. Long leg alignment views (*A*) and hind foot alignment views (*B*) of a 72-year-old woman presenting with a left-sided healed distal tibia fracture. There was a previous contralateral malunited proximal femoral fracture. The patient presented with an inability to mobilize because of tibial deformity, with pain at the malunion site and ankle.

of multifragmentary articular deformity, allowing for planning of fragment-specific osteotomy. Furthermore, the correction can be rehearsed and even implant positioning planned. Single-photon emission CT is used by some to gain more information regarding the asymmetrical loading of the ankle joint. MRI is useful in cases where assessment of the health of cartilage or suspected avascular necrosis.

Blood markers are unreliable when assessing for infection. If the clinical history is suggestive of such, then a multidisciplinary approach involving a microbiologist is essential. If there is any doubt, ankle joint aspiration, or bony biopsy, should be considered before undertaking reconstructive surgery. MRI is too sensitive and not specific, regarding the assessment of bony infection. White cell–labeled scans and single-photon emission CT are used,[12] but in our unit we have found that the use of fluorodeoxyglucose PET-CT is sensitive and specific when identifying the infected zones within the bone.

Broadly speaking, correction can occur at one of three levels: (1) correction of the mechanical axis in the metaphysis/supramalleolar region, (2) in the periarticular zone (including correction of joint incongruity), or (3) in the hindfoot. Careful clinical evaluation and review of imaging determines the level of the deformity and the most effective means of correcting this (**Fig. 4**). Radiographic deformity analysis is routinely undertaken using image manipulation software (eg, TraumaCad, Brainlab,

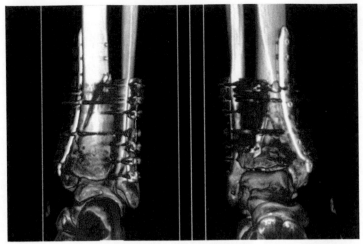

Fig. 2. 3D CT reconstruction with surface rendering allowing an appreciation of fracture fragment position and previous fracture planes.

Westchester, IL; Bone Ninja, International Center for Limb Lengthening, Baltimore, MD). The Baltimore Group have provided a pneumonic, or *aide-mémoire* for deformity assessment: MAP the ABCs (**Box 1**).[13]

CORRECTION OF THE MECHANICAL AXIS

The most common indications for a supramalleolar osteotomy are asymmetric valgus or varus osteoarthritis with at least 50% preserved tibiotalar joint surface.[14] However, ankle malunion causing post-traumatic asymmetrical loading of the ankle has widely been recognized as causing degenerative disease.[15,16] The supramalleolar osteotomy procedure is primarily concerned with congruent ankle joints (tibiotalar tilt <4°),

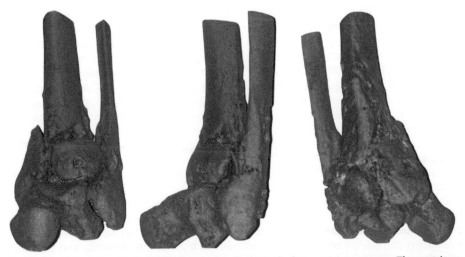

Fig. 3. 3D printed model of a malunited pilon fracture before revision surgery. The previous metal work has been digitally removed.

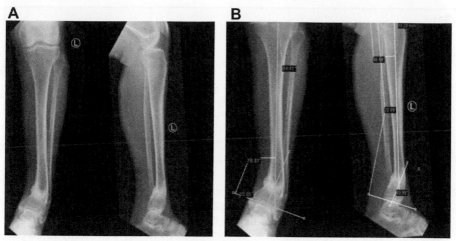

Fig. 4. (A) Picture demonstrates the pre-operative anteroposterior and lateral radiographs of the deformity of patient previously described in fig. 1. (B) Picture illustrates the mapping of the CORA onto these images.

although an additional procedure to the articular block can expand these indications.[17,18] Although coronal plane deformity is the most common indication, correction of tibial recurvatum deformity is also described.[19] Isolated corrective fibular osteotomies are indicated for some ankle malunions with some reporting the talus remaining tilted in up to 37% of fractures, with up to 50% of these patients subsequently developing osteoarthritis.[20,21] Hintermann and colleagues[22] reported in 48 malunited ankle fractures that additional realignment osteotomy of the tibia achieved 87.5% good or excellent results at 7 years with ongoing talus tilt only occurring in 10%.

The position of the osteotomy in relation to the center of rotation of angulation (CORA) and the nature of the osteotomy performed influence the way the bone heals during the correction phase. There are two scenarios where complete appreciation of the osteotomy rules (**Box 2**) is vital:

1. The CORA may be within the joint. It is not feasible to perform and intra-articular osteotomy; therefore, the osteotomy is performed in a safe anatomic location, as

---

Box 1

Aide-mémoire for deformity assessment: MAP the ABCs

This analysis should answer the questions: Is there a deformity? Which bone segment is deformed? Where is the apex of the deformity?

M – Measure the mechanical axis deviation

A – Analyze the joint angles

P – Pick the deformity

A – Apex of deformity (the center of rotation of angulation)

B – Bone cut (the level of the osteotomy)

C – Correction, either acute, or gradual

Data from Standard S, Herzenberg J, Conway J, Lamm B, Siddiqui N. *The art of limb alignment.* Baltimore, MD: Rubin Institute for Advanced orthopedics, Sinai Hospital of Baltimore; 2014.

Box 2
Osteotomy rules

1. When the osteotomy and angulation correction axis (ACA) pass through any of the CORAs, realignment occurs without translation.
2. When the ACA is through the CORA, but the osteotomy is performed at a different level than the CORA, the axis of the segments realigns by angulation with translation.
3. When the osteotomy and ACA are at a level above or below the CORAs the proximal and distal axes of the bone are parallel, but a translational deformity is created.

---

   close as possible to the apex of the deformity such that it affords bone fixation with adequate stability.
2. It may not be practical to perform the osteotomy at the level of the CORA, perhaps because of bone quality post-fracture healing, which would result in suboptimal bone regenerate formation. Alternatively, the soft tissue envelope, which may be scarred, would not be amenable to dissection to allow the osteotomy to be performed, compromising blood flow around the area and again having a negative effect on the healing of the osteotomy.

An osteotomy away from the CORA engenders translation, the extent of which is determined at the planning stage and whether or not this is acceptable. Some translation on occasion may be beneficial, in that it allows affected zones of the ankle joint to be offloaded. This is explained when the following is considered: deformity correction occurs about a bisector line at the CORA, a line that bisects the obtuse angle of the deformity. The axis about which the correction occurs is the angulation correction axis. Depending on whether the correction occurs on the convex, concave, or in the center of this determines if there is some shortening, or lengthening associated with the correction.

Level of Osteotomy

Choosing the appropriate level of osteotomy for a specific deformity optimizes outcomes (**Box 3**). Ultimately, correction of the deformity needs to be made, providing good alignment, optimizing bone contact, held with stable fixation that allows stimulation of healing (weight-bearing at an appropriate time), and with minimal biologic compromise. When the level of the osteotomy has been determined, the technique used to perform the osteotomy should be considered, how the correction is going to be performed, whether the correction is going to be performed gradually or acutely, and the hardware required to maintain the reduction.

The osteotomy is performed in several ways depending on surgeon preference. However, the method selected should ensure minimal thermal necrosis of bone, preserving biology and allowing bone healing. For transverse division of the bone, there are numerous descriptions of how to perform the osteotomy. These include Ilizarov corticotomy,[23] Gigli saw osteotomy,[24] and the De Bastiani osteotomy.[25] Each method of dividing the bone has its own idiosyncrasies (eg, a Gigli saw osteotomy is well suited to rotational correction). We have developed the Liverpool Method, a modification of the De Bastiani method, which involves three passes of a 4.8-mm cooled drill, down the lateral face of the tibia, the medial face, and one additional pass between. Then, a Hibbs osteotome is used first down the lateral face, then the medial face, and sequentially across the posterior aspect of the tibia. We find this a reliable and reproducible osteotomy, producing good regenerate bone. A latency of 7 to 10 days postosteotomy is built into the correction phase, allowing initial callus to form.[26]

Box 3
Relevant conditions to consider for the choice of appropriate level of osteotomy for a specific deformity

- Supramalleolar osteotomy:
  - Asymmetric disease with a varus or valgus component, allowing correction of distal tibia deformity following fracture
  - Minimal talar tilt
  - Can be combined with intra-articular osteotomy
  - Hindfoot realignment before, or with joint sacrificing procedures

- Periarticular osteotomy
  - Distal tibial oblique osteotomy for asymmetric ankle osteoarthritis
  - Plafond-plasty
  - Fibular osteotomy

- Intra-articular
  - Tibial plafond incongruity following fracture

Internal Fixation Supramalleolar Osteotomies

Correction of distal tibial deformities is most commonly undertaken acutely, requiring incisions for the osteotomy and use of internal hardware. Several authors have highlighted the importance of skin bridges greater than 7 cm between two approaches around the ankle to reduce the risk of soft tissue complications.[27,28] Howard and colleagues[29] argued in their approaches study on pilon fractures, skin bridges 5 cm could be tolerated with low wound complication rates. Previous skin scars and adherent soft tissue preclude some approaches. Gradual correction of a deformity may be preferable in some scenarios, such as where soft tissues do not allow for acute correction, or when the characteristics of the patient are not suitable. This is most predictably achieved using an external fixator.

In acute corrections, a valgus deformity is most commonly performed using a medial closing wedge. For varus deformity correction, a medial opening (**Fig. 5**) or lateral closing osteotomy (**Fig. 6**) are commonly indicated, with the lateral closing wedge osteotomies preferred in larger deformities (varus deformity >10°) to prevent subfibular impingement.[30–32] Nha and colleagues[33] performed a cadaveric study looking at the safe zone for supramalleolar osteotomy. To prevent complete osteotomy, and preserve the lateral cortical hinge, they recommended that the osteotomy was placed in plane with the proximal one-third of the syndesmosis.[33] Kim and colleagues[34] supported these findings, with no changes in ankle motion found in supra-syndesmotic compared with intrasyndesmotic osteotomy. Ettinger and colleagues[35] biomechanical study tested five different implants in opening wedge supramalleolar osteotomy and found all performed well with no significant difference for failure load. Several authors have reported favorable mid- to long-term outcomes, with low rate of conversion to ankle fusion/replacement.[16,30,36]

A dome osteotomy is used for the correction of coronal plane deformity of the distal tibia. In comparison with alternative open, or closing wedge osteotomy techniques, it allows scope for a massive correction, without the disadvantages of needing bone graft, or shortening the tibia (**Fig. 7**). The osteotomy center of rotation is planned at the center of the deformity. The radius of the osteotomy is produced using a plate as a compass,[36] or alternatively using a distal tibia circular frame five-hole rancho cube[37] or a half pin with a three-hole rancho (**Fig. 8**). Once the osteotomy of the tibia and fibula have been performed, adjustable correction is possible until the planned degree of correction is achieved. The nature of the

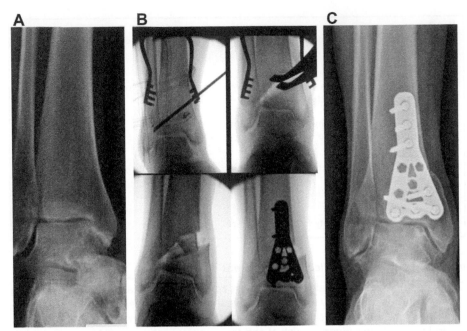

Fig. 5. (A) Post-traumatic medial osteoarthritis with medial bone-on-bone contact, widening of the ankle mortise and vertical medial malleolus. The central images (B) show the intraoperative radiographs with preplanned insertion of an osteotome to create a distal tibial oblique osteotomy allowing the lateral hinge to occur intrasyndesmotic. A laminar spreader is used to correct the tibial-articular angulation followed by insertion of iliac crest autograft and fixation. (C) Postoperative weight-bearing radiograph with improved articular congruency.

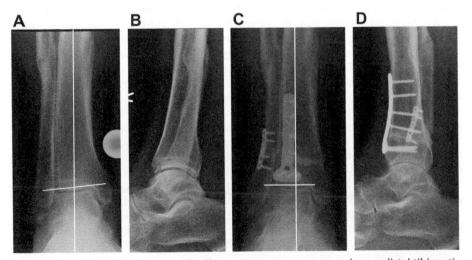

Fig. 6. (A, B) Preoperative radiographs illustrating a procurvatum and varus distal tibia articular alignment as a consequence of a previous tibial malunion. (C, D) Postoperative radiographs illustrating a lateral closing wedge tibial osteotomy and fibular osteotomy with correction of articular alignment. Because of the osteotomy being made away from the CORA, lateral translation has occurred.

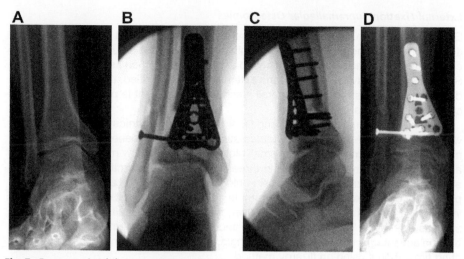

Fig. 7. Preoperative (*A*), intraoperative (*B, C*), and postoperative (*D*) imaging of a right ankle with significant varus deformity treated with a dome osteotomy.

osteotomy means that it cannot pass directly through the CORA, so translation will occur. The main benefit of the dome is the reliable bone contact, which confers good stability and predictable bone healing at the osteotomy. Rosteius and colleagues[38] reported good short-term outcomes in a small series of large deformities corrected using dome osteotomy.

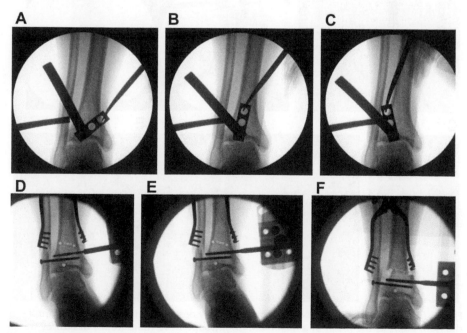

Fig. 8. (*A–C*) Three-hole rancho with guide inserted over a half-pin, with the radius of the osteotomy being demonstrated. (*D, E*) Dome osteotomy and fibular osteotomy with the application of an LRS advanced rail medially, with a swivel clamp applied to allow correction. (*F*) Correction before fixation.

External Fixation Supramalleolar Osteotomies

External fixators are routinely used in either temporarily assisting correction or definitively correcting and stabilizing a deformity. Temporary assisted correction is more commonly performed using an inline mono external fixator, such as the LRS Advanced Rail (Orthofix, Lewisville, TX). Once the external fixator is applied, the osteotomy is undertaken, an assessment of the overall mechanical alignment is performed, and then correction proceeds.

In definitive deformity correction and fixation, the biomechanics of a tensioned finewire external fixator should not be underestimated. Its main benefits are the result of minimal soft tissue insult, leaving a small biologic footprint, early mobilization, and the ability to correct large deformities in three dimensions. Deformity is corrected with either traditional Ilizarov methods, using hinges and motors, or alternatively a hexapod. In our own personal experience, simple deformities are most easily corrected using the Ilizarov method (**Fig. 9**). If, however, the deformity is multiplanar, a hexapod, such as the Taylor Spatial Frame (Smith and Nephew, Inc, Memphis, TN) (**Fig. 10**), has the advantages of potentially producing a more compact frame, in a shorter operating time, than if using an Ilizarov method.

Consideration needs to be made to the position of the rings relative to the planned level of the osteotomy and the safe corridors for passage of wires and half-pins.[39] The shape of the frame proximal to the osteotomy depends on the characteristics of the patient and the device used. There is usually space for only one ring distal to the

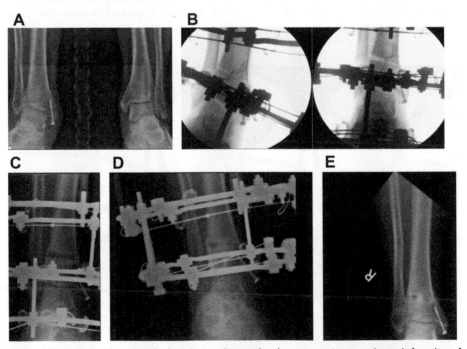

Fig. 9. (A) Comparative weight-bearing radiographs demonstrating a valgus deformity of the right ankle as the result of a malunion. (B) Intraoperative radiographs of Ilizarov frame application and osteotomy. The rings have been set on either side of the osteotomy such that they are orthogonal to their respective bone segments. (C) Acute correction of the deformity with a lateral opening wedge. (D, E) Healing of the osteotomy, preframe and post-frame removal.

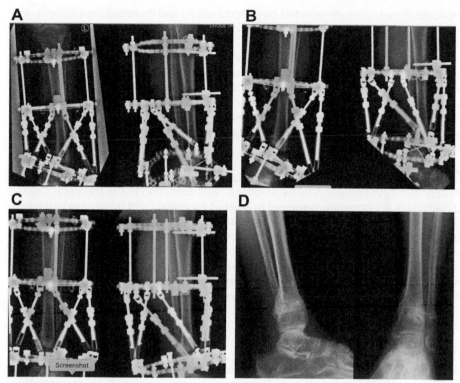

Fig. 10. (*A*) Postoperative radiograph of patient from **Fig. 1** with application of a Taylor Spatial Frame. Note the osteotomy between ring 2 and 3 is just distal to the CORA (the fracture site). Osteotomy at the CORA would have been through sclerotic united bone, which would have produced unreliable callus. (*B*) About 10 mm of distraction to allow angular correction. (*C*) Angular adjustment is now complete, with sagittal and coronal alignment correction. (*D*) Completion of treatment with correction of the tibial mechanical axis.

osteotomy because of the proximity to the talocrural joint line. It is therefore common to bridge the ankle during the correction phase, for added stability, and the heel ring can be removed at 6 to 8 weeks post-frame application.

CORRECTION OF INTRA-ARTICULAR DEFORMITY

Ankle incongruency is in combination or isolated to mechanical axis deviation following pilon or ankle malunion. Chao and colleagues[40] commented that the most important factor in the development of valgus malunion was rotation and shortening of the fibula. The medial ligaments become attenuated, allowing lateral deviation and tilt. Conversely, persistent lateral ligament instability results in unbalanced loading of the medial tibial plafond.[41] Mann and colleagues[41] described the medial malleolus to be no longer vertical, with a medially inclined articulation, thanks to the impact of the talus, which is driven medially.

Plafond-Plasty

Mann and colleagues[41] described an opening medial tibial wedge osteotomy (plafond-plasty) in 19 patients, using an intra-articular CORA, with 15 out of 18 being either satisfied or very satisfied with their treatment. Hintermann and colleagues[18] could not replicate the early results reported on plafond-plasty and therefore developed a double tibia osteotomy, an intra-articular opening wedge and medial tibia opening wedge osteotomy. This allowed a significantly greater deviation of the weight-bearing axis laterally as plafond-plasty alone. At an average of 5.9 years, the results in 20 patients showed a significant improvement in pain and function, with VAS pain improving from 7.9 ± 1.3 to 1.3 ± 1.6 and American Orthopaedic Foot and Ankle Society hindfoot score from 49 ± 15 point to 86 ± 12 points.[18] Guo and colleagues also reported on combined plafond-plasty with supramalleolar osteotomy, in 24 patients with malunited medial impacted ankle fractures. They reported results equivalent to the previous paper in pain and function.[42]

Fibula Osteotomy

Fibular malunion correction by osteotomy is well described in the literature. Oblique osteotomies are generally described to correct shortening and minimal external rotation (<10°) and transverse osteotomies are described to correct malunions with greater external rotation.[31,32,40,43] More complex Z osteotomies have also been reported to lengthen the fibular.[44] The outcomes reported in the literature postfibular osteotomy are generally good, with van Wensen and colleagues[32] finding in a literature review of 177 patients, good or excellent outcomes in 77%. Chao and colleagues[40] reported in 12 patients no radiographic evidence of arthritis progression at mean 30 months postosteotomy. The main factor thought to negatively influence the clinical outcome is preexisting arthritis.[41]

Intra-Articular Step-Off

Ankles have a significantly higher incidence of post-traumatic arthritis as compared with other weight-bearing joints.[45] The unique anatomic and cellular characteristics of the articular cartilage within the ankle joint make it more susceptible to post-traumatic osteoarthritis.[46] Persistent postoperative step-off of the ankle articular surface has been reported to have higher incidence of post-traumatic osteoarthritis. Verhage and colleagues[47] found in their study in posterior malleolar fractures, a persistent step-off of greater than 1 mm was the greatest risk factor (odds ratio, 4.16; 95% confidence interval, 1.50–11.57) for development of osteoarthritis. Revision of malunited or healing malreductions involve careful planning. 3D CT reconstruction is imperative to understand each fracture plane (**Figs. 11** and **12**) and the use of 3D printed models allows the planning and practice of the case before completion. 3D printed patient-specific surgical guides have been studied by Weigelt and colleagues[48] who reported promising results. Previous scars and immobile soft tissues can limit exposure and it is imperative that the integrity of any potential skin bridges and their angiosomes are assessed before surgery.

ADDITIONAL PROCEDURES

On history, examination, and operative planning the necessity to perform procedures in addition to the correction of extra-articular or intra-articular deformity need to be considered. Frequently, however, the requirement for additional surgery can only be assessed at time of operation. Several authors have reported a high incidence of additional procedure requirement with distal tibia osteotomies.[18,22,30,42,49] The nature of the osteotomy in itself may result in returning the correct tension to supporting ligaments enabling congruency of the mortise joint, but additional ligament reconstruction may be required.[18,30] Hintermann and colleagues[18] noted the most common additional procedure to be a lateral ligament reconstruction in 70% of double

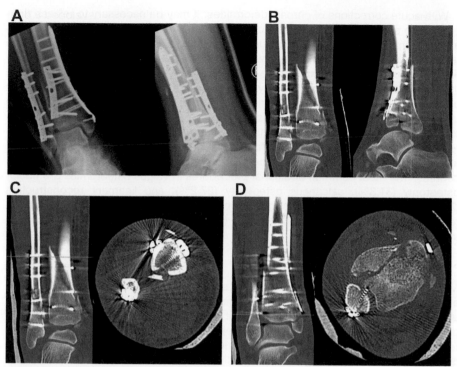

Fig. 11. (*A*) Plain AP and Lateral radiographs and (*B-D*) CT imaging of a complex malreduced pilon fracture. The radiographs although difficult to interpret show an elevated anterior plafond and a double joint line shadow on the AP radiograph. The CT confirms these findings.

osteotomies of the distal tibia. Guo and colleagues[33] reported that they routinely performed anterior drawer testing and varus stress radiographs during the operation. If the angle of the tibiotalar tilt on the varus stress anteroposterior radiograph was more than 9° or if the anterior displacement on the anterior drawer lateral radiograph was more than 10 mm, they performed a lateral ligament reconstruction.

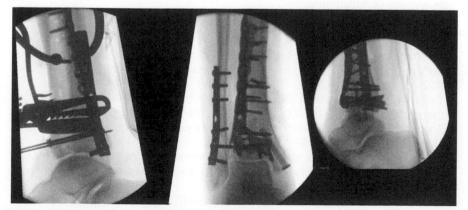

Fig. 12. Intraoperative image intensifier images illustrating revision of the malreduced pilon from **Fig. 11**, with removal of previous metal work and osteotomy through fracture planes.

With acute corrections of chronic deformities, it may be necessary to release tight soft tissue structures, such as the Achilles tendon, to allow for sufficient correction and realignment of the hindfoot. Guo and colleagues[42] commented that Achilles tendon contractures were assessed with the heel in neutral position and the knee in extension followed by the knee in flexion to isolate and address the contracture at the time of surgery. Osteophytes may also require debridement to return joint range of motion, with Scheidegger and colleagues[19] reporting a 46% cheilectomy of the talus neck in tibial flexion osteotomies.

Additional bony procedures of the calcaneum, midfoot, and forefoot may be required to achieve a plantar grade foot.[18,49,50] Krähenbühl and colleagues[30] noted a different percentage of additional procedures in valgus compared with varus procedures. The most common additional procedures in valgus osteotomies are fibular osteotomy (31.3%), calcaneus osteotomy (27.2%), and ligament reconstruction (22.1%). In varus procedures the most common additional procedures are ligament reconstruction (42.4%), fibular osteotomy (33.3%), and peroneus longus to brevis transfer (22.2%).[30]

SUMMARY

Malunion of ankle and pilon fractures has significant detrimental effect on function and development of post-trauma osteoarthritis. Unfortunately, the incidence of malunion has been reported to be increasing. It is important to assess the ankle for congruency, because this determines the level where correction occurs. A plethora of techniques are available, with low-level evidence supporting each, and therefore it is important that the treating surgeon is fully prepared and comfortable in the techniques they are to use. Supplementary procedures are common and should be expected.

DISCLOSURE

Mr L.W. Mason is a paid consultant with implant companies, Stryker and Orthosolutions. Mr L.W. Mason is an implant designer for Orthosolutions.

ACKNOWLEDGMENT

The authors thank Dr Andy Molloy and Dr Durai Nayagam for their contribution to the article and use of radiographs.

REFERENCES

1. Mauffrey C, Vasario G, Battiston B, et al. Tibial pilon fractures: a review of incidence, diagnosis, treatment, and complications. Acta Orthop Belg 2011;77(4): 432–40.
2. Dujardin F, Abdulmutalib H, Tobenas AC. Total fractures of the tibial pilon. Orthop Traumatol Surg Res 2014;100(1 Suppl):S65–74.
3. Topliss CJ, Jackson M, Atkins RM. Anatomy of pilon fractures of the distal tibia. J Bone Joint Surg Br 2005;87(5):692–7.
4. Wei SJ, Han F, Lan SH, et al. Surgical treatment of pilon fracture based on ankle position at the time of injury/initial direction of fracture displacement: a prospective cohort study. Int J Surg 2014;12(5):418–25.
5. Zhang SB, Zhang YB, Wang SH, et al. Clinical efficacy and safety of limited internal fixation combined with external fixation for Pilon fracture: A systematic review and meta-analysis. Chin J Traumatol 2017;20(2):94–8.

6. Zelle BA, Dang KH, Ornell SS. High-energy tibial pilon fractures: an instructional review. Int Orthop 2019;43(8):1939–50.
7. Whitehouse S, Mason LW, Jayatilaka L, et al. Fixation of ankle fractures - a major trauma centre's experience in improving quality. Ann R Coll Surg Engl 2019; 101(6):387–90.
8. Roberts V, Mason LW, Harrison E, et al. Does functional outcome depend on the quality of the fracture fixation? Mid to long term outcomes of ankle fractures at two university teaching hospitals. Foot Ankle Surg 2019;25(4):538–41.
9. Saltzman CL, el-Khoury GY. The hindfoot alignment view. Foot Ankle Int 1995; 16(9):572–6.
10. Lintz F, Welck M, Bernasconi A, et al. 3D biometrics for hindfoot alignment using weightbearing CT. Foot Ankle Int 2017;38(6):684–9.
11. Lal H, Patralekh MK. 3D printing and its applications in orthopaedic trauma: a technological marvel. J Clin Orthop Trauma 2018;9(3):260–8.
12. Arican P, Okudan B, Sefizade R, et al. Diagnostic value of bone SPECT/CT in patients with suspected osteomyelitis. Mol Imaging Radionucl Ther 2019;28(3): 89–95.
13. Standard S, Herzenberg J, Conway J, et al. The art of limb alignment. Baltimore (MD): Rubin Institute for Advanced Orthopedics; 2014.
14. Ewalefo SO, Dombrowski M, Hirase T, et al. Management of posttraumatic ankle arthritis: literature review. Curr Rev Musculoskelet Med 2018;11(4):546–57.
15. Thordarson DB, Motamed S, Hedman T, et al. The effect of fibular malreduction on contact pressures in an ankle fracture malunion model. J Bone Joint Surg Am 1997;79(12):1809–15.
16. Stufkens SA, Knupp M, Lampert C, et al. Long-term outcome after supination-external rotation type-4 fractures of the ankle. J Bone Joint Surg Br 2009; 91(12):1607–11.
17. Knupp M, Stufkens SA, Bolliger L, et al. Classification and treatment of supramalleolar deformities. Foot Ankle Int 2011;32(11):1023–31.
18. Hintermann B, Ruiz R, Barg A. Novel double osteotomy technique of distal tibia for correction of asymmetric varus osteoarthritic ankle. Foot Ankle Int 2017; 38(9):970–81.
19. Scheidegger P, Horn Lang T, Schweizer C, et al. A flexion osteotomy for correction of a distal tibial recurvatum deformity: a retrospective case series. Bone Joint J 2019;101-B(6):682–90.
20. Marti RK, Raaymakers EL, Nolte PA. Malunited ankle fractures. The late results of reconstruction. J Bone Joint Surg Br 1990;72(4):709–13.
21. Offierski CM, Graham JD, Hall JH, et al. Late revision of fibular malunion in ankle fractures. Clin Orthop Relat Res 1982;171:145–9.
22. Hintermann B, Barg A, Knupp M. Corrective supramalleolar osteotomy for malunited pronation-external rotation fractures of the ankle. J Bone Joint Surg Br 2011;93(10):1367–72.
23. Schwartsman V, Schwartsman R. Corticotomy. Clin Orthop Relat Res 1992;(280): 37–47.
24. Paktiss AS, Gross RH. Afghan percutaneous osteotomy. J Pediatr Orthop 1993; 13(4):531–3.
25. De Bastiani G, Aldegheri R, Renzi-Brivio L, et al. Limb lengthening by callus distraction (callotasis). J Pediatr Orthop 1987;7:129–34.
26. GA I. Transosseous osteosynthesis: theoretical and clinical aspects of the regeneration and growth of tissue. Softcover reprint of the hardcover. 1st edition. Springer-Verlag; 1992.

27. Thordarson DB. Complications after treatment of tibial pilon fractures: prevention and management strategies. J Am Acad Orthop Surg 2000;8(4):253–65.

28. Bonar SK, Marsh JL. Tibial plafond fractures: changing principles of treatment. J Am Acad Orthop Surg 1994;2(6):297–305.

29. Howard JL, Agel J, Barei DP, et al. A prospective study evaluating incision placement and wound healing for tibial plafond fractures. J Orthop Trauma 2008;22(5): 299–305 [discussion: 305–96].

30. Krahenbuhl N, Zwicky L, Bolliger L, et al. Mid- to long-term results of supramalleolar osteotomy. Foot Ankle Int 2017;38(2):124–32.

31. Egger AC, Berkowitz MJ. Operative treatment of the malunited fibula fracture. Foot Ankle Int 2018;39(10):1242–52.

32. van Wensen RJ, van den Bekerom MP, Marti RK, et al. Reconstructive osteotomy of fibular malunion: review of the literature. Strateg Trauma Limb Reconstr 2011; 6(2):51–7.

33. Nha KW, Lee SH, Rhyu IJ, et al. Safe zone for medial open-wedge supramalleolar osteotomy of the ankle: a cadaveric study. Foot Ankle Int 2016;37(1):102–8.

34. Kim HJ, Yeo ED, Rhyu IJ, et al. Changes in ankle joint motion after Supramalleolar osteotomy: a cadaveric model. BMC Musculoskelet Disord 2017;18(1):389.

35. Ettinger S, Schwarze M, Yao D, et al. Stability of supramalleolar osteotomies using different implants in a sawbone model. Arch Orthop Trauma Surg 2018;138(10): 1359–63.

36. Colin F, Gaudot F, Odri G, et al. Supramalleolar osteotomy: techniques, indications and outcomes in a series of 83 cases. Orthop Traumatol Surg Res 2014; 100(4):413–8.

37. Chatterton BD, Bing A. A novel technique for supramalleolar osteotomy of the tibia using a circular frame. Ann R Coll Surg Engl 2019;101(5):373–4.

38. Rosteius T, Baecker H, Schildhauer TA, et al. Correction of posttraumatic deformities of the distal tibia with focal dome osteotomy. Unfallchirurg 2018;121(12): 976–82 [in German].

39. Nayagam S. Safe corridors in external fixation: the lower leg (tibia, fibula, hindfoot and forefoot). Strateg Trauma Limb Reconstr 2007;2(2–3):105–10.

40. Chao KH, Wu CC, Lee CH, et al. Corrective-elongation osteotomy without bone graft for old ankle fracture with residual diastasis. Foot Ankle Int 2004;25(3): 123–7.

41. Mann HA, Filippi J, Myerson MS. Intra-articular opening medial tibial wedge osteotomy (plafond-plasty) for the treatment of intra-articular varus ankle arthritis and instability. Foot Ankle Int 2012;33(4):255–61.

42. Guo C, Liu Z, Xu Y, et al. Supramalleolar osteotomy combined with an intra-articular osteotomy for the reconstruction of malunited medial impacted ankle fractures. Foot Ankle Int 2018;39(12):1457–63.

43. Henderson WB, Lau JT. Reconstruction of failed ankle fractures. Foot Ankle Clin 2006;11(1):51–60, viii.

44. Weber D, Friederich NF, Muller W. Lengthening osteotomy of the fibula for posttraumatic malunion. Indications, technique and results. Int Orthop 1998;22(3): 149–52.

45. Brown TD, Johnston RC, Saltzman CL, et al. Posttraumatic osteoarthritis: a first estimate of incidence, prevalence, and burden of disease. J Orthop Trauma 2006;20(10):739–44.

46. Kraeutler MJ, Kaenkumchorn T, Pascual-Garrido C, et al. Peculiarities in ankle cartilage. Cartilage 2017;8(1):12–8.

47. Verhage SM, Krijnen P, Schipper IB, et al. Persistent postoperative step-off of the posterior malleolus leads to higher incidence of post-traumatic osteoarthritis in trimalleolar fractures. Arch Orthop Trauma Surg 2019;139(3):323–9.
48. Weigelt L, Furnstahl P, Hirsiger S, et al. Three-dimensional correction of complex ankle deformities with computer-assisted planning and patient-specific surgical guides. J Foot Ankle Surg 2017;56(6):1158–64.
49. Deforth M, Krahenbuhl N, Zwicky L, et al. Supramalleolar osteotomy for tibial component malposition in total ankle replacement. Foot Ankle Int 2017;38(9):952–6.
50. Barg A, Pagenstert GI, Horisberger M, et al. Supramalleolar osteotomies for degenerative joint disease of the ankle joint: indication, technique and results. Int Orthop 2013;37(9):1683–95.

Managing Severely Malunited Calcaneal Fractures and Fracture-Dislocations

Stefan Rammelt, MD, PhD*, Christine Marx, MD

KEYWORDS

- Calcaneus • Malunion • Nonunion • Necrosis • Peroneal tendon dislocation
- Ankle impingement • Osteotomy • Fusion

KEY POINTS

- Severe calcaneal malunions are debilitating conditions owing to severe hindfoot deformity with painful subtalar arthritis and soft tissue impingement.
- Type III malunions with substantial loss of height are best treated with a subtalar distraction bone block fusion and additional osteotomies in case of severe varus or superior displacement of the calcaneal tuberosity.
- Type IV malunions with lateral and cranial shift of the calcaneal body result from malunited calcaneal fracture-dislocations and require a 3-dimensional corrective osteotomy along the former fracture plane.
- Type V malunions with talar tilt warrant additional ankle debridement and reconstruction of the calcaneal shape to provide support for the talus in the ankle mortise.
- Accompanying soft tissue procedures include Achilles tendon lengthening, peroneal tendon release, and rerouting behind the lateral malleolus.

INTRODUCTION: PATHOMECHANISM OF THE DEFORMITY

Malunions of the calcaneus are a common source of severe pain and disability. They are caused by nonoperative treatment and inadequate reduction and/or fixation of displaced calcaneal fractures and fracture-dislocations.[1–4] Consequently, the features of calcaneal malunions reflect the original fracture mechanism. The axial impact of the initial fracture mechanism leads to direct cartilage damage, a loss of height, and widening of the calcaneus.[5–7] The typical bulging of the lateral wall impinges the peroneal tendons and the fibular tip. With severe deformity, this may cause a chronic dislocation of the tendons and deformity of the distal fibula.[1,8,9] Intra-articular step-offs and

---

University Hospital Carl Gustav Carus, TU Dresden, Fetscherstrasse 74, Dresden 01307, Germany
* Corresponding author. University Center for Orthopaedics and Traumatology, University Hospital Carl Gustav Carus, TU Dresden, Fetscherstrasse 74, Dresden 01307, Germany.
E-mail address: strammelt@hotmail.com

Foot Ankle Clin N Am 25 (2020) 239–256
https://doi.org/10.1016/j.fcl.2020.02.005
1083-7515/20/© 2020 Elsevier Inc. All rights reserved.

incongruity result in subtalar and calcaneocuboid arthritis.[10] Unrecognized sustentacular fractures result in a loss of medial support of the talus and secondary varus deformity.[11,12] The eccentric pull of the Achilles tendon adds to the bony shortening, varus or valgus malalignment of the hindfoot.[3,13]

With severe deformity of the calcaneus, talar inclination, and sometimes even talar tilting in the ankle mortise owing to the loss of calcaneal support leads to an anterior ankle impingement and arthritis.[1,13,14] These conditions have a negative impact on foot function because hindfoot deformity and loss of motion affect the adjacent joints, that is, the ankle and mid tarsal joints, that are essential for normal function. Restriction of movement, an inability to walk on uneven ground, conflict with regular footwear, and nerve irritations are common.

To improve foot function, decrease pain and conflict with shoe wear, minimize soft tissue impingement, and prevent arthritis of adjacent joints, realignment of the hindfoot with correction of the deformity is warranted. Joint-preserving osteotomies are used in rare cases of extra-articular malunions or intra-articular malunions without symptomatic arthritis.[15–17] Regularly, manifest arthritis of the subtalar joint will be present at the time of patient presentation and deformity correction has to be combined with subtalar fusion. This may be achieved with asymmetric joint resection, structural bone grafting, additional corrective osteotomy of the calcaneus, and revision of the ankle joint in the most severe deformities.[1,3,9,10,13,18–20]

PATIENT ASSESSMENT

Surgical correction of severe calcaneal malunions is challenging and needs to be adapted to the patients' individual soft tissue conditions, comorbidities, functional demand, and compliance. Preoperative assessment requires a thorough analysis of the whole lower limb, including the previously uninjured side. Because the post-traumatic deformity is a direct consequence of the initial fracture pathoanatomy, it should always be attempted to recall the original mechanism of injury.

The lower leg is inspected for any visible deformities. The foot is inspected for scars and callosities, the latter pointing to eccentric loading and hidden deformities or imbalances. The ankle, subtalar, and midtarsal joints are examined for range of motion, crepitus, and stability. The affected leg has to be evaluated for adequate circulation and sensation as well as muscle power and balance. If circulation seems to be inadequate, Doppler studies or angiography should be performed before major reconstruction is planned. Besides the foot itself, inspection of regularly worn shoes and insoles are most valuable in evaluating the mechanical consequences of longstanding deformities.[21]

Radiographic examination includes anteroposterior weight-bearing radiographs of the ankle, anteroposterior (dorsoplantar), and lateral weight-bearing radiographs of the whole foot (**Fig. 1**) and a hindfoot alignment of long axial view for any suspected axial deviation.[22,23] The most important measure in both the lateral view and dorsoplantar view is the talus-first metatarsal axis (Meary's line).[24] Other useful measures for planning hindfoot corrections are the talar declination angle (which directly affects the talus-first metatarsal axis), calcaneal pitch angle, talocalcaneal height, navicular-to-floor distance, and cuboid-to-floor distance.[25,26] Furthermore, as in acute calcaneal fracture treatment, Böhler's (tuberosity joint) and Gissane's (crucial) angles are important measures, if still discernible in complex malunions. The formerly uninjured foot serves as a reference for correction.

For complex deformities, computed tomography scanning is generally advised for 3-dimensional planning of the corrective surgery (**Fig. 2**).[1] The extent of post-traumatic

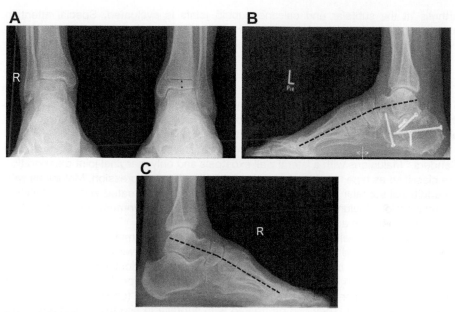

Fig. 1. Standing anteroposterior (A) and lateral (B) radiographs of a 76-year-old man presenting 13 years after minimally invasive screw fixation of a comminuted calcaneal fracture because of an initial wound infection. The main feature is a considerable loss of calcaneal height (type III deformity). Note the talar inclination and subsequent anterior ankle impingement on the left side. (C) The formerly uninjured side that serves as a template for correction has an intrinsic cavus deformity with a talus-first metatarsal angle of 10°. It is 15° on the symptomatic left side.

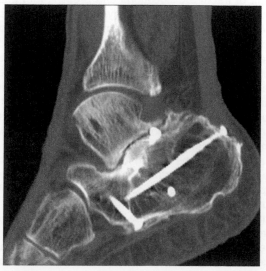

Fig. 2. A computed tomography scan of the same patient as in Fig. 1 shows a severe narrowing of the subtalar joint space and partially intra-articular screw position.

arthritis at the subtalar and calcaneocuboid joints is evaluated. Special attention should be paid to the presence of nonunion, avascular necrosis or signs of a local infection. In cases of doubt, MRI, bone scan, and laboratory examinations may be indicated.

CLASSIFICATION AND PLANNING

The 3-dimensional correction of severely malunited calcaneal fractures requires a thorough preoperative analysis of the deformity. Currently used classification systems allow tailoring of the operative treatment to the type of deformity.

The first classification for calcaneal malunions was provided by Stephens and Sanders.[3] Malunions with a lateral wall exostosis and only marginal joint deterioration are classified as type I and treated with a lateral wall decompression. Malunions with an additional subtalar arthritis are classified as type II and treated with an additional subtalar fusion. Malunions with an additional varus malalignment are classified as type III and need an additional Dwyer osteotomy.[27]

Zwipp and Rammelt[1] distinguished 5 types of calcaneal malunions[13] and a sixth type has been added later. Type 0 refers to any deformity without the presence of arthritis. These may be extra-articular or selected intra-articular malunions, which may be treated with a joint-preserving osteotomy.[15,16] Type I malunions present with a painful subtalar arthritis but without relevant deformity (equivalent to Stephens and Sanders Type II). They can be treated with subtalar in situ fusion and additional lateral wall decompression as needed. Type II resembles Stephens and Sanders type III deformities, with additional varus or valgus malalignment of the hindfoot. These deformities require an asymmetric joint resection, fusion with wedge shaped bone blocks or additional osteotomy of the tuberosity. A synopsis of these classifications is provided in **Fig. 3**.

Type III malunions represent the typical deformity after calcaneal fractures with an additional loss of height resulting in a decreased or reversed Böhler's angle. The classical treatment consists of a subtalar bone block distraction fusion.[18,26,28] In case of severe malalignment, an additional osteotomy may become necessary. Type IV malunions are the result of fracture dislocations and present with a lateral and cranial translation of the tuberosity and calcaneal body. This further results in a painful fibulocalcaneal abutment and chronic dislocation/impingement of the peroneal tendons. Two-part fracture dislocations of the calcaneus are rare and can be overlooked easily, because the shape of the calcaneus seems to be intact in the lateral radiographic view.[5,29] These deformities require a 3-dimensional corrective osteotomy along the former fracture plane with subtalar fusion.[1,20] Type V malunions represent the most severe deformity and are characterized by an additional talar tilt in the ankle mortise. This condition results from a complex deformity with loss of support of the talus from the calcaneus. Consequently, in addition to these measures, an open revision of the ankle joint and corrective subtalar fusion is needed.[9,13]

In general, calcaneal malunions should be corrected as early as possible after detection because post-traumatic arthritis in the subtalar joint develops rapidly and will prevent joint-sparing corrections in most cases.[15] Furthermore, long-standing severe deformities of the calcaneus will result in eccentric loading and subsequent arthritis of adjacent joints, most notably the ankle and mid tarsal joints, which are all essential for normal foot function.[13]

Correction of the bony deformities is typically accompanied by additional procedures for soft tissue balancing, such as lateral wall decompression, tenolysis, and rerouting of the peroneal tendons with reconstruction of the superior peroneal retinaculum, and lengthening of the Achilles tendon.[1]

Stephens/ Sanders classification	Zwipp/Rammelt classification	Characteristics	Treatment options
Type 1 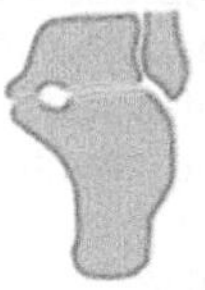	Type 0 Any malunion without subtalar arthritis	Lateral exostosis, joint cartilage intact	Exostosectomy, lateral wall decompression, joint-preserving osteotomy
Type 2 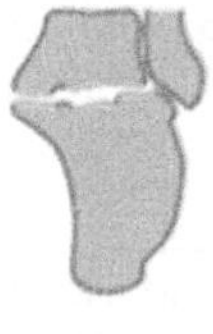	Type I arthritis 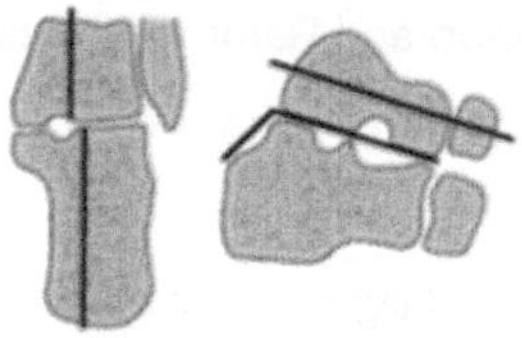	Arthritis of the subtalar joint	In situ fusion of the subtalar joint
Type 3 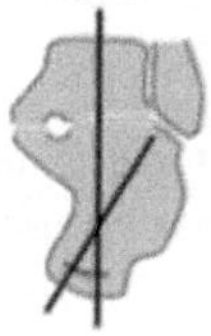	Type II + varus/valgus 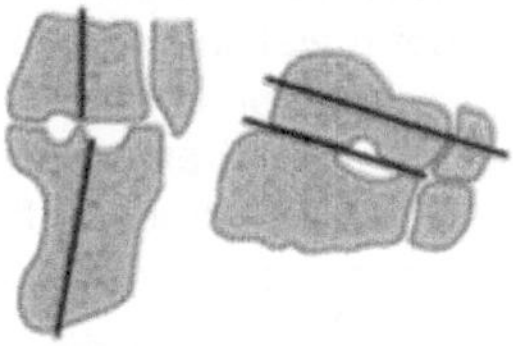	Additional hindfoot varus/ valgus	Corrective subtalar fusion (asymmetric joint resection, osteotomy, bone block fusion)
	Type III + loss of height 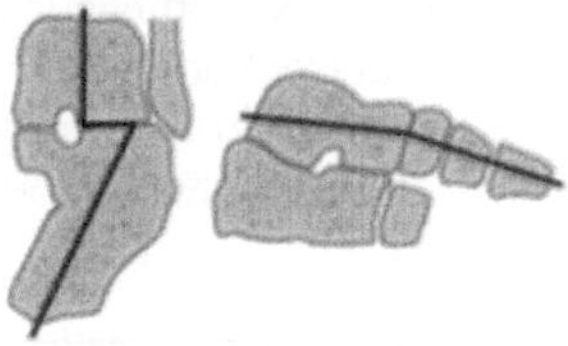	Additional loss of heel height	Subtalar bone block distraction fusion, additional osteotomy for severe deformity
	Type IV + lateral translation 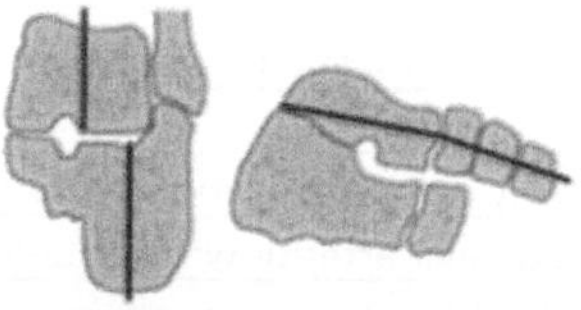	Lateral and upward translation of the tuberosity (malunited fracture-dislocation)	Corrective osteotomy along the former fracture with subtalar fusion and bone grafting
	Type V + talar tilt 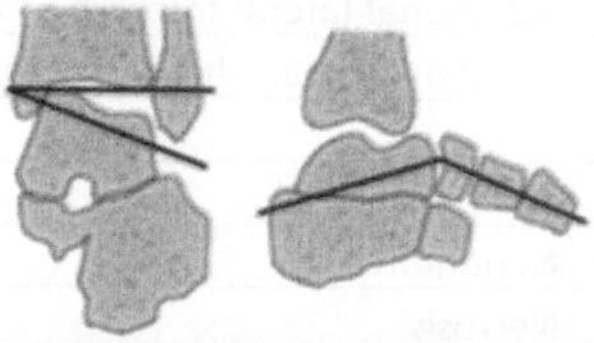	Irregular deformity with deep impaction of the talus into the calcaneus with secondary tilt in the ankle mortise	Corrective osteotomy/fusion, ankle revision, ligament balancing

Fig. 3. Synopsis of the Stephens and Sanders and Zwipp and Rammelt classifications for calcaneal malunions with proposed treatment options. (*From* Sanders RW, Rammelt S. Fractures of the Calcaneus. In: Coughlin MJ, Saltzman CR, Anderson JB, eds. Mann's Surgery of the Foot & Ankle. 9th Ed, Philadelphia, PA: Elsevier Saunders; 2014: 2041-2100; with permission.)

The treatment of all types of malunions may be further complicated by the presence of a nonunion or avascular necrosis. For classification purposes, the quality of the bony malunion can be labeled with additional letters. Subtype A stands for a solid malunion, B for nonunion, and C for osteonecrosis. In case of a nonunion, all fibrous and sclerotic tissue is resected until viable bone becomes visible. Avascular necrosis requires a radical debridement of all nonviable bone. In both cases, the defect needs to be filled with autograft or allograft at the time of correction. A lingering infection needs to be ruled out by multiple biopsies. If chronic infection is suspected, a staged protocol of serial debridements with secondary reconstruction once negative results from swabs and biopsies are obtained is implemented.

A summary of treatment options is provided in **Table 1**. We concentrate on the correction of severe deformities, that is, Zwipp and Rammelt types 3 to 5.

CORRECTION OF TYPE III MALUNIONS
Subtalar Distraction Bone Block Fusion

Arthritis of the subtalar joint, varus or valgus malalignment of the hindfoot, and a loss of calcaneal height are the most common consequences of nonoperative treatment or inadequate reduction and/or fixation of displaced, intraarticular calcaneal fractures. These type III malunions show a typical hindfoot malalignment with reduced or even reversed Böhler's angle, talar inclination with anterior tibiotalar impingement and therefore an increased risk of subsequent arthritis of the ankle joint (see **Figs. 1** and **2**). The treatment of choice is a subtalar bone block distraction fusion that corrects the loss of height and has a certain potential of correcting varus or valgus deformity via the size and shape of the bone blocks used.[14,19]

If no lateral calcaneal plate has to be removed, a posterolateral (Gallie) approach to the subtalar joint is preferred because it provides a good soft tissue cover and avoids tension at the wound edges even with substantial correction of the heel height.[19,26] In addition, the wedge-shaped bone blocks are introduced much easier from the back than from the front. The patient is placed prone and a longitudinal skin incision lateral

Table 1
Classification of post-traumatic malunions

	Characterization of Malunion
Type	
0	Any deformity without arthritis
I	Subtalar arthritis without deformity
II	Additional varus or valgus
III	Additional loss of height
IV	Additional lateral translation of the tuberosity
V	Additional talar tilt
Quality	
A	Solid malunion
B	Nonunion
C	Necrosis

Modified from Zwipp H, Rammelt S. Posttraumatic deformity correction at the foot. Zentralbl Chir 2003;128(3):218-226 and Rammelt S, Zwipp H. Corrective arthrodeses and osteotomies for post-traumatic hindfoot malalignment: Indications, techniques, results. Int Orthop. 2013;37(9):1707-17; with permission.

and parallel to the Achilles tendon is carried out. Care is taken to spare the sural nerve that is running in the subcutaneous tissue from the midline toward the lateral aspect of the calcaneus. The superficial and deep fascia are incised longitudinally. The flexor hallucis longus muscle is mobilized and its tendon protects the posterior tibial neurovascular bundle that is held away medially. The peroneal tendons are retracted laterally. After dissection of the posterior capsule the subtalar joint is identified. In case of large posterior osteophytes and gross deformity it may be wise to locate the subtalar joint under fluoroscopy to avoid debridement at the posterior aspect of the ankle joint. After correct identification of the subtalar joint, all residual cartilage and sclerotic bone is removed with chisels, burrs, and curettes. A laminar spreader is used to distract the joint and the surrounding soft tissues after complete debridement. The correction and the amount of bone grafting needed for correction of the physiologic axes at the foot are then checked fluoroscopically (**Fig. 4**).

A Schanz screw that is inserted percutaneously into the calcaneal tuberosity or a collinear pin distractor between the tip of the fibula and the tuberosity may be helpful to achieve stepwise the desired realignment, especially with long-standing, severe deformities. Additional lengthening of the Achilles tendon is often required because of shortening of the triceps surae.[1] This procedure may be carried out as a percutaneous Z-plasty. The surgeon has to decide individually if a complete correction of the deformity is to be achieved, or if a slight undercorrection is accepted to reduce strain on the soft tissue envelope, particularly in the presence of severe scarring.

After the desired realignment of the hindfoot has been achieved, the calcaneus is fixed temporarily to the talus with Kirschner wires. The exact required size of the bone blocks is measured. Two tricortical bone blocks are harvested from the ipsilateral posterior iliac crest and inserted under press fit. Alternatively, allografts of the desired size may be used. A slight varus or valgus is corrected with differently sized bone blocks. Two 6.5-mm screws are introduced percutaneously from the posterior calcaneal tuberosity into the talar body (**Fig. 5**). Depending on good bone quality, partially threaded screws are used as lag screws; for poor bone stock, fully threaded screws are used as set screws. Alternatively, cannulated screws may be used.

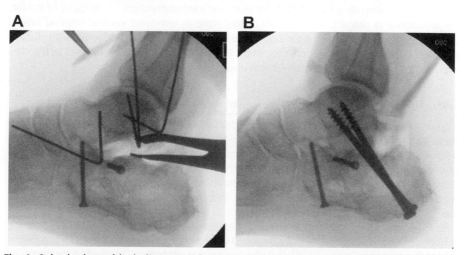

Fig. 4. Subtalar bone block distraction fusion in the same patient as in **Figs. 1** and **2**. (*A*) After removing the posterior screws and joint debridement, heel height is restored using a laminar spreader. (*B*) Realignment requires 2 bone blocks of 2 cm. Fixation is achieved with screws.

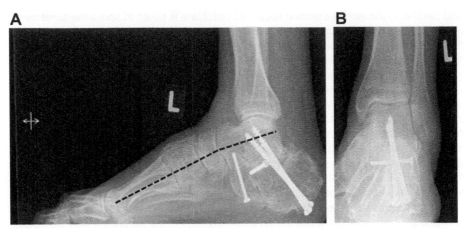

Fig. 5. One-year follow-up of the same patient as in **Figs. 1, 2, and 4** showing bony consolidation of the subtalar bone block distraction fusion. (*A*) Heel height and talus-first metatarsal axis are restored to the values of the formerly uninjured side. Anterior tibiotalar impingement is released. (*B*) The anteroposterior view shows physiologic valgus of the heel.

In case of previous calcaneal fracture fixation with a lateral plate, the healed lateral scar is used and the implants are removed first. For that, the patient is placed in a lateral decubitus position. In the case of severe bulging of the lateral calcaneal wall, removal of the plate and lateral wall decompression leaves enough room for tension-free wound closure at the end of the corrective surgery.[8] The lateral wall of the calcaneus is decompressed with a chisel and the soft tissue is protected. Typically, the peroneal tendons have to be freed from adhesions and impingement on the tendons will be released by decompressing the bulged lateral wall of the calcaneus. If a large piece of bone has to be removed for excessive bulging of the lateral wall, it can be used as a bone block for subtalar joint distraction.[8,10] In case of doubt, the procedure is staged. In a first step, the plate is removed via the original lateral approach. In a second step, after complete wound healing, corrective subtalar fusion is carried out via a posterolateral approach, which is more or less equivalent to the vertical limb of the original extensile lateral approach.[30,31]

Subtalar Distraction Bone Block Fusion with Additional Osteotomy

In type III malunions with substantial axial deviation, hindfoot alignment in the coronal plane cannot be achieved with asymmetric joint resection or shaping of the bone blocks. In particular, with severe varus deformity of the heel, the pull of the deltoid ligament will prevent excessive correction through the joint.[3,26] In these cases, an additional closing wedge osteotomy of the calcaneal tuberosity in the coronal plane is needed to correct severe hindfoot varus deformity. The removed wedge may be used for subtalar joint distraction.

Similarly, in case of excessive upward displacement of the tuberosity with inversion of Böhler's angle, a craniocaudally directed osteotomy is needed to correct the deformity of the calcaneal body.[9,16,21,32] A closing wedge osteotomy is needed for complex deformities (**Fig. 6**). If of adequate size and bone quality, the resected wedge may be used for subtalar joint distraction, thus avoiding additional harvesting of bone graft (**Figs. 7 and 8**).[33]

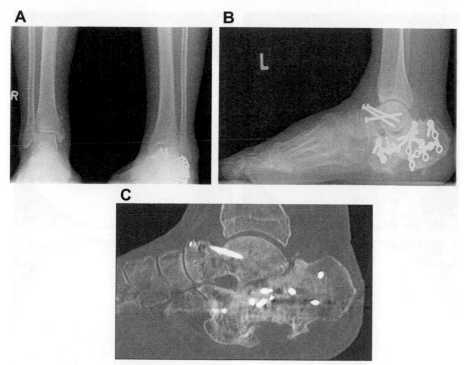

Fig. 6. A 67-year-old, active man presents with increasing pain in the lateral heel 2.5 years after operative treatment of a complex fracture of the talus and calcaneus. (*A*) Anteroposterior and (*B*) lateral radiographs show substantial loss of height and varus deformity of the heel. The calcaneal plate is broken and the (*C*) computed tomography scan confirms severe subtalar arthritis as well as sclerotic bone in the subthalamic area but no signs of nonunion.

Typically, calcaneocuboid arthritis does not become symptomatic in a substantial number of cases. Only in cases of painful arthritis of the calcaneocuboid joint, it should be fused using an oblique lateral approach (lateral utility)[21] or an existing extensile lateral approach. If a type III malunion is complicated by a nonunion or avascular necrosis, all fibrous, sclerotic, or necrotic tissue is debrided and additional cancellous bone grafting is used to obtain bony consolidation.[1]

CORRECTION OF TYPE IV MALUNIONS

In type IV malunions with a lateral and cranial displacement of the calcaneal body (**Fig. 9**A, B), the 3-dimensional correction can be achieved via an oblique sliding osteotomy along the former primary fracture line.[1,9,20] A slightly curved anterolateral approach is used as in acute calcaneal fracture-dislocations.[29] The skin incision starts over the lateral malleolus and is continued over the sinus tarsi toward the anterior calcaneal process. Care must be taken not to injure the peroneal tendons that are chronically dislocated into the subcutaneous tissue over the tip of the fibula. The tendons are freed from adhesions and then mobilized caudally and held away with a soft strap. The fibrous tissue between the tip of the fibula and the displace calcaneal tuberosity is debrided and a laminar spreader is introduced between them. Alternatively, a femoral distractor is placed between the calcaneal tuberosity and the tibia.

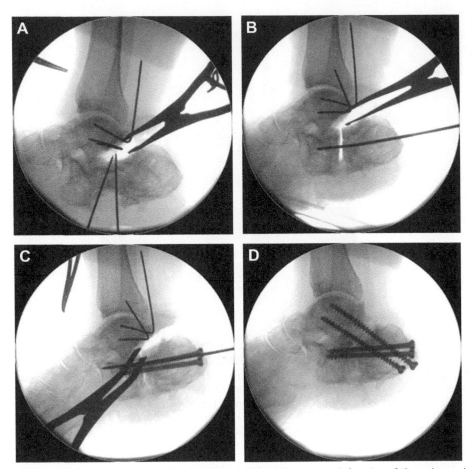

Fig. 7. (*A*) Subtalar distraction alone does not correct the severe deformity of the calcaneal body. (*B*) An additional closing wedge osteotomy at the calcaneal body is performed to lower the tuberosity. (*C*) The osteotomy is fixed with screws. (*D*) The resected bone wedge is used as bone block for the subtalar distraction fusion. In addition, the screws from the talus were removed because they contributed to anterior ankle impingement (same patient as in **Fig. 6**).

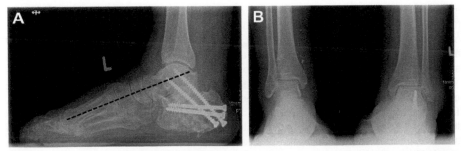

Fig. 8. (*A*, *B*) Standing radiographs 12 weeks postoperatively demonstrate physiologic hind-foot alignment and bony consolidation (same patient as in **Figs. 6** and **7**).

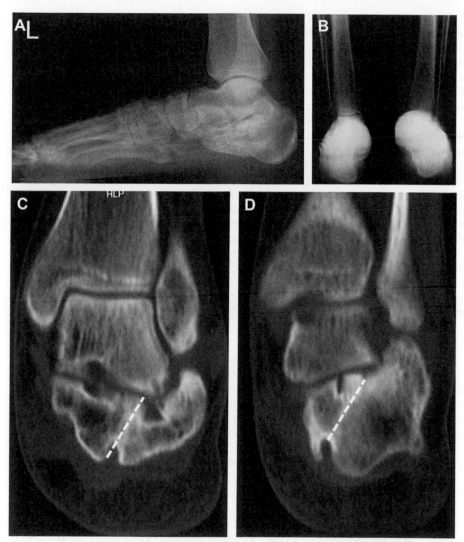

Fig. 9. Malunited calcaneal fracture-dislocation (type IV deformity) in a 48-year-old man. (*A*) Note the double contour in the lateral radiograph and the (*B*) lateral and upward displacement of the calcaneal body in the axial view. (*C*) Computed tomography scanning reveals a solid malunion along the former primary fracture (*interrupted line*) that serves as the plane for the corrective osteotomy. (*D*) Typically, upward and lateral shift of the calcaneal body results in painful fibulocalcaneal abutment and chronic dislocation of the peroneal tendons, which are displaced from the fibular groove.

The former fracture line is identified as a large stepoff in the subtalar joint, which is debrided. Typically, the joint cartilage is still present over the medial aspect of the subtalar joint that is still in its physiologic position. Very rarely, in simple 2-part fracture dislocations that are not very old, the cartilage remains intact over the lateral aspect of the subtalar joint. In these cases, the osteotomy can be carried out with joint preservation.[15] Typically, at the time of presentation, the joint cartilage is gone and severe subtalar arthritis is present (**Fig. 9**C, D). After joint debridement, the osteotomy is carried out with a chisel following the former fracture line that may be marked with Kirschner wires from superolateral to inferomedial. Care is taken not to Injure the tibial neurovascular bundle that may run close to the medial exit of the former fracture. In case of excessive scarring, an additional medial approach may be performed beneath the sustentaculum tali. The tibial neurovascular bundle is carefully mobilized with the flexor halluces longus tendon. The deep trough in the medial calcaneal wall is then easily identified and can be used to guide the osteotomy.

After completion of the osteotomy, correction of the calcaneal body fragment is carried out gradually by using an elevator between the main fragments, a laminar spreader between the fibula and calcaneus, a Schanz screw in the tuberosity, or a femoral distractor between the tibia and calcaneus.[1] This maneuver regularly requires an Achilles tendon lengthening. Once correction is achieved, it is held by a large point-to-point reduction forceps placed from the sustentaculum tali to the lateral calcaneal wall. Correct realignment is verified fluoroscopically and held temporarily with Kirschner wires. The main lateral fragment of the calcaneus is fixed against the sustentaculum and the medial wall with 4.5-mm (or 3.5-mm) lag screws (**Fig 10**). Any remaining defect at the subtalar joint level is filled with appropriately sized bone blocks from the iliac crest or cancellous bone. Alternatively, an allograft may be used. Subtalar fusion is achieved with screws from the posterior tuberosity into the talar body. After bony correction has been achieved, the peroneal tendons can be rerouted behind the lateral malleolus and the superior peroneal retinaculum is reconstituted.[1]

CORRECTION OF TYPE V MALUNIONS

In the most severe calcaneal malunions, the talus has completely lost its support because of a severe calcaneal depression and deformity.[13,14] In these rare cases, the talus not only displays an inclination in the sagittal plane, but also a varus tilt within the ankle mortise in the coronal plane (**Fig. 11**). These type V malunions require an additional anteromedial approach for debridement of the ankle joint from ingrown tissue and adhesions and to control the exact alignment of the talus within the ankle mortise after correction of the calcaneal deformity.[1]

After a 3-dimensional osteotomy of the calcaneus with restoration of its shape, the talus can be elevated. This maneuver may require an additional osteotomy and

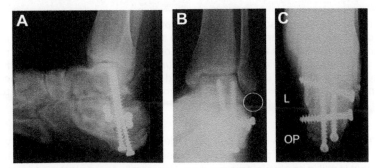

Fig. 10. (A–C) Salvage of malunited calcaneal fracture-dislocations consists of a corrective sliding osteotomy of the calcaneus along the former fracture plane and subtalar fusion with bone graft as needed (same patient as in **Fig. 9**). The horizontal screws stabilize the calcaneal osteotomy and the vertical screws hold the subtalar fusion. The fibulocalcaneal impingement is completely resolved; see the circle in (B).

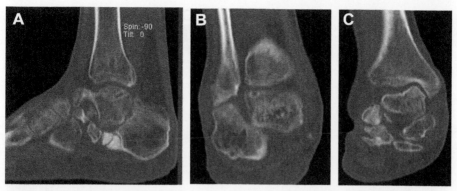

Fig. 11. (A–C) Type V malunion in a 47-year-old active man with a severe deformity of the calcaneus and subsequent talar tilt in the ankle mortise presenting 1.5 years after poly-trauma with serial injuries to the lower extremity sustained in a paragliding injury. An amorphous bone cement has been filled into the caudal aspect of the calcaneus without internal fixation.

stabilization of the anterior process of the calcaneus (**Fig. 12**). The talus is realigned in the ankle mortise and subtalar distraction fusion is performed as described elsewhere in this article. Any remaining defect from the calcaneal body needs to be filled with bone graft to maintain the support for the talus from the calcaneus (**Fig. 13**).

AFTER TREATMENT

After corrective bone block distraction fusion, a split below-knee cast or arthrodesis boot is fitted depending on patient conditions and complexity of surgery. Partial weight bearing up to 20 kg on 2 crutches is allowed in compliant patients. Patients gradually progress to full weight bearing after radiographic evidence of fusion

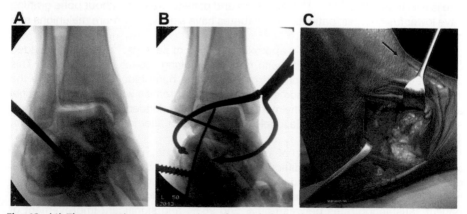

Fig. 12. (A) The corrective osteotomy is performed along the former fracture plane as in a type IV deformity using a curved lateral approach. Note the Schanz screw in the calcaneal tuberosity used for distraction. (B) The lateral (tuberosity/body) fragment is held against the sustentaculum with a point-to-point reduction clamp. (C) The position of the talus is controlled via an anterior approach to the ankle (*arrow*). After correction of the calcaneus, the peroneal tendons (held with a soft strap) can be rerouted behind the lateral malleolus (same patient as in **Fig. 11**).

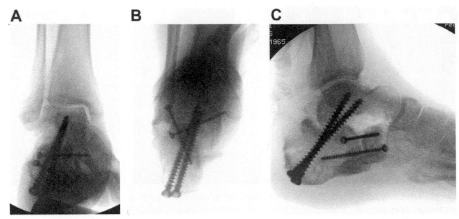

Fig. 13. (*A–C*) Subtalar distraction fusion was completed using a bicortical bone block from the iliac crest and 4.5-mm screws. This particular deformity also required a corrective osteotomy of the anterior calcaneal process. The calcaneocuboid joint could be preserved because there was sufficient cartilage cover on the calcaneal facet. Fixation of the calcaneal fragments was achieved with additional 3.5-mm screws (same patient as in **Figs. 11** and **12**).

(**Fig. 14**), typically at 12 weeks postoperatively. An intensive protocol of physical therapy is necessary to achieve a good compensatory range of motion in the ankle and midtarsal (Chopart) joints and a near normal gait. Implants are only removed if symptomatic.

RESULTS AND COMPLICATIONS

Nonunion of the subtalar fusion is a typical complication after corrective surgery for calcaneal malunion. In most of the series with greater patient numbers, the nonunion rate is less than 10%.[18,26,27,33–36] Smokers and patients treated without bone grafting have lower fusion rates; patients with diabetes have significantly more malunions and nonunions after subtalar fusion.[35]

Wound complications occur in approximately 6% of patients.[36] The most dreaded complication is a deep infection with osteitis requiring repeat debridements. This complication is usually accompanied by loss of the bone blocks. To eradicate the infection, the treating surgeon sometimes has to compromise with respect to the final amount of correction. Polymethylmethacrylate cement loaded with antibiotics may serve as a temporary spacer (Masquelet technique)[37] or alternatively as a permanent, stable implant.[38]

Owing to the great variety of calcaneal malunions, comparison of different studies from the literature is difficult. A substantial number of studies only exists on subtalar distraction bone block fusion for type III malunions with union rates between 86% and 100%, substantial correction of talocalcaneal height (5–11 mm), patient satisfaction rates between 50% and 96%, and significant improvement of the average functional scores as compared with the preoperative values.[1,18,19,26,27,33–36] Correction of radiographic parameters correlated well with the functional results including gait analysis and pedobarographic data in 2 studies.[26,34] Substantial improvement was also found in smaller case series for correction of malunited calcaneal fracture-dislocations (type IV and V malunions) via 3-dimensional osteotomies.[9,20]

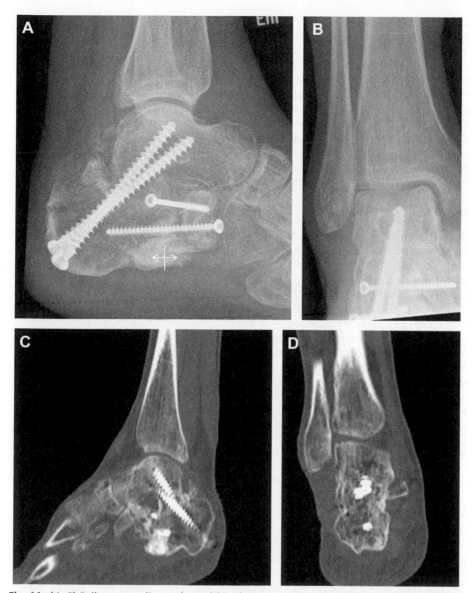

Fig. 14. (*A, B*) Follow-up radiographs and (*C, D*) computed tomography scans 9 months after correction showing bony consolidation without loss of correction (same patient as in **Figs. 11–13**).

Favorable results have also been reported for correction of calcaneal malunions following an individualized treatment algorithm tailored to the individual deformity.[1,3,8,9] However, patients have to be counseled that, owing to the complex deformity necessitating fusion of the subtalar joint and associated soft tissue pathologies, corrective procedures as described elsewhere in this article do not result in a full functional recovery of the severely injured foot.[26]

Fusion of an arthritic joint can alleviate pain, but has to be combined with deformity correction to regain reasonable foot function and protct adjacent joints.[1,19,26,34] In situ fusion of calcaneal malunions without correction of the deformity was associated with poor outcome and functional parameters were correlated to the degree of remaining deformity.[39] In contrast, owing to soft tissue restraints, corrective fusion for severe malunion is challenging and better functional outcomes with fewer wound complications were associated with subtalar fusion for the treatment of symptomatic post-traumatic subtalar arthritis after initial open reduction and internal fixation of a displaced intra-articular calcaneal fracture as compared with corrective subtalar arthrodesis for the treatment of calcaneal malunion after initial nonoperative treatment.[40] Initial open reduction and internal fixation of displaced, intra-articular calcaneal fractures restores calcaneal shape, alignment, and height, which facilitates a secondary fusion procedure if needed and establishes an opportunity to achieve a better long-term functional result.[4,6,41]

SUMMARY

Severe calcaneal malunions result from inadequate treatment of intra-articular calcaneal fractures and fracture-dislocations. They are debilitating conditions owing to severe hindfoot deformity with painful subtalar arthritis, eccentric loading of adjacent joints, soft tissue imbalance, and impingement. Type III malunions with substantial loss of height are treated with a subtalar distraction bone block fusion. Additional osteotomies may be required for severe varus or superior displacement of the calcaneal tuberosity. Type IV malunions, that is, malunited calcaneal fracture-dislocations, with lateral and cranial shift of the calcaneal body require a 3-dimensional corrective osteotomy along the former fracture plane. Type V malunions with talar tilt warrant additional ankle debridement and reconstruction of the calcaneal shape to provide support for the talus in the ankle mortise. Bony reconstruction is regularly accompanied by soft tissue balancing. The most frequent procedures include Achilles tendon lengthening, peroneal tendon release, and rerouting behind the lateral malleolus for chronic dislocation owing to calcaneofibular abutment.

REFERENCES

1. Rammelt S, Zwipp H. Corrective arthrodeses and osteotomies for post-traumatic hindfoot malalignment: indications, techniques, results. Int Orthop 2013;37(9): 1707–17.
2. Sangeorzan BJ, Hansen ST Jr. Early and late posttraumatic foot reconstruction. Clin Orthop Relat Res 1989;243:86–91.
3. Stephens HM, Sanders R. Calcaneal malunions: results of a prognostic computed tomography classification system. Foot Ankle Int 1996;17:395–401.
4. Rammelt S, Sangeorzan BJ, Swords MS. Calcaneal fractures – should we or should we not operate? Indian J Orthop 2018;52:220–30.
5. Rammelt S, Bartoníček J, Park KH. Traumatic injury to the subtalar joint. Foot Ankle Clin 2018;23(3):353–74.
6. Sanders R, Vaupel ZM, Erdogan M, et al. Operative treatment of displaced intra-articular calcaneal fractures: long-term (10-20 Years) results in 108 fractures using a prognostic CT classification. J Orthop Trauma 2014;28(10):551–63.
7. Ball ST, Jadin K, Allen RT, et al. Chondrocyte viability after intra-articular calcaneal fractures in humans. Foot Ankle Int 2007;28(6):665–8.
8. Clare MP, Lee WE 3rd, Sanders RW. Intermediate to long-term results of a treatment protocol for calcaneal fracture malunions. J Bone Joint Surg Am 2005;87(5): 963–73.

9. Zwipp H, Rammelt S. Subtalar arthrodesis with calcaneal osteotomy. Orthopade 2006;35(4):387–404.
10. Sanders RW, Rammelt S. Fractures of the calcaneus. In: Coughlin MJ, Saltzman CR, Anderson JB, editors. Mann's surgery of the foot & ankle. 9th edition. Philadelphia: Elsevier Saunders; 2013. p. 2041–100.
11. Dürr C, Zwipp H, Rammelt S. Fractures of the sustentaculum tali. Oper Orthop Traumatol 2013;25(6):569–78.
12. Rammelt S, Pitakveerakul A. Hindfoot injuries: how to avoid post-traumatic varus deformity? Foot Ankle Clin 2019;24:325–45.
13. Zwipp H, Rammelt S. Posttraumatic deformity correction at the foot. Zentralbl Chir 2003;128:218–26.
14. Carr JB. Varus of the talus in the ankle mortise secondary to calcaneus fracture. A case report. Clin Orthop Relat Res 1991;263:206–9.
15. Rammelt S, Grass R, Zwipp H. Joint-preserving osteotomy for malunited intra-articular calcaneal fractures. J Orthop Trauma 2013;27(10):e234–8.
16. Ketz J, Clare M, Sanders R. Corrective osteotomies for malunited extra-articular calcaneal fractures. Foot Ankle Clin 2016;21(1):135–45.
17. Benirschke SK, Kramer PA. Joint-preserving osteotomies for malaligned intraarticular calcaneal fractures. Foot Ankle Clin 2016;21(1):111–22.
18. Carr JB, Hansen ST, Benirschke SK. Subtalar distraction bone block fusion for late complications of os calcis fractures. Foot Ankle 1988;9(2):81–6.
19. Klaue K, Hansen ST. Principles of surgical reconstruction of the mid- and hindfoot. Foot Ankle Surg 1994;1:37–44.
20. Romash MM. Reconstructive osteotomy of the calcaneus with subtalar arthrodesis for malunited calcaneal fractures. Clin Orthop 1993;290:157–67.
21. Rammelt S, Hansen ST, Zwipp H. Posttraumatic reconstruction of the foot and ankle. In: Browner BD, Jupiter JB, Krettek C, et al, editors. Skeletal trauma. 6th edition. Philadelphia: Elsevier Saunders; 2019. p. 2641–90.
22. Saltzman CL, El-Khoury GY. The hindfoot alignment view. Foot Ankle Int 1995; 16(9):572–6.
23. Reilingh ML, Beimers L, Tuijthof GJ, et al. Measuring hindfoot alignment radiographically: the long axial view is more reliable than the hindfoot alignment view. Skeletal Radiol 2010;39(11):1103–8.
24. Meary R. Le pied creux essentiel. Rev Chir Orthop Reparatrice Appar Mot 1967; 53(5):389–410.
25. Buch BD, Myerson MS, Miller SD. Primary subtalar arthrodesis for the treatment of comminuted calcaneal fractures. Foot Ankle Int 1996;17(2):61–70.
26. Rammelt S, Grass R, Zawadski T, et al. Foot function after subtalar distraction bone-block arthrodesis. A prospective study. J Bone Joint Surg Br 2004;86(5): 659–68.
27. Dwyer FC. Osteotomy of the calcaneum for pes cavus. J Bone Joint Surg Br 1959;41(1):80–6.
28. Trnka HJ, Easley ME, Lam PW, et al. Subtalar distraction bone block arthrodesis. J Bone Joint Surg Br 2001;83(6):849–54.
29. Rammelt S, Zwipp H. Fractures of the calcaneus: current treatment strategies. Acta Chir Orthop 2014;81:177–96.
30. Letournel E. Open treatment of acute calcaneal fractures. Clin Orthop Relat Res 1993;290:60–7.
31. Rammelt S, Zwipp H. Calcaneus fractures: facts, controversies and recent developments. Injury 2004;35(5):443–61.

32. Huang PJ, Fu YC, Cheng YM, et al. Subtalar arthrodesis for late sequelae of calcaneal fractures: fusion in situ versus fusion with sliding corrective osteotomy. Foot Ankle Int 1999;20(3):166–70.
33. Kassem MS, Elgeidi A, Badran M, et al. Sagittal resection osteotomy with bone block distraction subtalar fusion for treatment of malunited calcaneal fractures. J Foot Ankle Surg 2019;58(4):739–47.
34. Farouk A, Ibrahim A, Mokhtar M, et al. Effect of subtalar fusion and calcaneal osteotomy on function, pain, and gait mechanics for calcaneal malunion. Foot Ankle Int 2019;40(9):1094–103.
35. Chahal J, Stephen DJ, Bulmer B, et al. Factors associated with outcome after subtalar arthrodesis. J Orthop Trauma 2006;20(8):555–61.
36. Schepers T. The subtalar distraction bone block arthrodesis following the late complications of calcaneal fractures: a systematic review. Foot (Edinb) 2013; 23(1):39–44.
37. Masquelet A, Kanakaris NK, Obert L, et al. Bone repair using the Masquelet technique. J Bone Joint Surg Am 2019;101(11):1024–36.
38. Qiu XS, Zheng X, Shi HF, et al. Antibiotic-impregnated cement spacer as definitive management for osteomyelitis. BMC Musculoskelet Disord 2015;16:254.
39. Ågren PH, Tullberg T, Mukka S, et al. Post-traumatic in situ fusion after calcaneal fractures: a retrospective study with 7-28 years follow-up. Foot Ankle Surg 2015; 21(1):56–9.
40. Radnay CS, Clare MP, Sanders RW. Subtalar fusion after displaced intra-articular calcaneal fractures: does initial operative treatment matter? J Bone Joint Surg Am 2009;91(3):541–6.
41. Rammelt S, Zwipp H, Schneiders W, et al. Severity of injury predicts subsequent function in surgically treated displaced intraarticular calcaneal fractures. Clin Orthop Relat Res 2013;471:2885–98.

The Use of Virtual Planning and Patient-specific Guides to Correct Complex Deformities of the Foot and Ankle

Stephan H. Wirth, MD[a], Norman Espinosa, MD[b],*

KEYWORDS

- Patient-specific guides • Osteotomy • Virtual • Planning

KEY POINTS

- Virtual planning software helps determine the type of deformity.
- Virtual analysis software helps plan the corrective surgery.
- Due to this technology, highly accurate corrections can be achieved.
- Virtual planning and transformation into in vivo correction are time efficient and might reduce the risk of potential complications.
- The costs related to this technology are reasonable.

INTRODUCTION

Foot and ankle surgeons are often confronted with complex deformities, which pose difficulties in finding an optimal means of correction. This is strongly connected to the identification of the so-called center of rotation of angulation (CORA).[1] The more complex the deformity, the harder to find the CORA; thus, it also is more difficult to achieve a proper correction.

In order to identify the magnitude of deformity, imaging modalities have become a standard tool in the preoperative analysis. Conventional radiographs, computed tomography (CT), magnetic resonance imaging (MRI), and even single-photon emission computer tomography (SPECT) help depict the pathologies and plan surgical interventions more precisely. Traditionally, however, preoperative planning of corrective osteotomies have been done based on 2-dimensional radiographs or certain CT slides extracted from the whole CT databases.[1] This is a fundamental

[a] Department of Orthopaedics, University of Zurich, The Balgrist, Forchstrasse 340, Zurich 8008, Switzerland; [b] Institute for Foot and Ankle Reconstruction, Fussinstitut Zurich, Kappelistrasse 7, Zurich 8002, Switzerland
* Corresponding author.
E-mail address: espinosa@fussinstitut.ch

Foot Ankle Clin N Am 25 (2020) 257–268
https://doi.org/10.1016/j.fcl.2020.02.004
1083-7515/20/© 2020 Elsevier Inc. All rights reserved.

error: a correction cannot be achieved by simple addition of 2-dimensional measurement modalities.[2]

The true 3-dimensional (3-D) correction angle can be estimated using planar measurements.[3] A deformity is always 3-D, including not only angular but also translational and rotational components. Therefore, an accurate correction of deformity can be achieved only when all components are seen in a 3-D environment, allowing the tackling of each of them properly.[2,3]

The data obtained in CT and/or MRI allow full 3-D information gathering. In addition, those imaging modalities provide a means of exact measurement of angular deformities and identification of the optimal osteotomy line. Schweizer and coworkers[4] published their methodology in order to virtually simulate any osteotomy in a computer.

This article discusses the advances that have been made in recent years regarding virtual planning and execution of complex osteotomies in the treatment of major deformities around the foot and ankle.[5]

BASIC TECHNOLOGICAL ASPECTS

In the treatment of unilateral deformities, it has been shown that the use of radiographs and/or CT of the contralateral healthy side could serve as a template for reconstruction.[6,7] Based on this simple planning, however, it remains difficult to ascertain intraoperatively whether the preoperative planned correction could be achieved. This is due to lack of specific verifying tools. Some centers provide an intraoperative CT scanner, which enables an immediate check of the surgical result. Although small alterations might be assessed by this tool, it is extremely difficult to find the optimal surgical solution to improve the overall result during the procedure.

Assisting systems, so-called smart tools or intraoperative navigation (REF), have had limited success and have not found widespread use in daily orthopedic practice. Systems for intraoperative navigation are expensive and difficult to handle. Thus, a surgeon continues to depending on experience, 2-dimensional planning tools, and manual measurement techniques to manage the surgery.

Based on those known problems, the authors were involved in the development of a computer-based planning tool, CASPA (Balgrist CARD AG, Zurich, Switzerland), that enabled analyzing deformities in a most accurate manner, to plan the surgery as precisely as possible while providing the technology to produce patient-specific guides for the intervention.[4,8,9]

INDICATIONS

Indications for the use of this specific correction tool (CASPA) encompass any deformity of the foot, ankle, tibia, and fibula. A majority of cases comprise posttraumatic and extra-articular deformities. Rotational and angular misalignments as well as length discrepancies can be addressed and corrected. Currently, the most preferred deformities for planning are unilateral ones, because the contralateral healthy side is used as a 3-D template in order to reconstruct and restore normal anatomy. In patients with bilateral, other templates need to be found, for example, a patient's leg axis or templates of already stored normal legs.

TECHNIQUE

In order to use the technique of virtual planning with CASPA, it is necessary to obtain a full set of CT data concerning the involved extremity as well as the healthy side. These data are used to generate a 3-D computer model by segmentation technique.[10]

Segmentation is achieved by identifying the cortical information (density according to measured gray values on CT scans), which is then separated from the surrounding anatomic structures. Contemporary and commercially available segmentation software (Mimics; Materialise, Leuven, Belgium) and semiautomatic segmentation algorithms (thresholding and region growing) allow quick and easy preparation of the data within minutes.[11,12]

The next step is to render a 3-D model of the surface. The complex surface of the bone is filled with triangular elements and thus mathematically replaced. By so doing, the pathologic and healthy bone shapes are arranged and ready for use for the 3-D analysis and surgical planning.[5,13]

To allow precise planning, the healthy bone is mirrored and used as template for correction. Both bones are perfectly aligned onto each other. In cases of a misaligned bone after fracture, the model can be divided into 3 parts: the fracture area, a proximal nondeformed area, and a distal nondeformed area around the fracture area. Using registry methodology, like iterative closed point, the proximal bone parts of both the healthy and pathologic bones are laid over each other.[14] A computerized model then is automatically applied and iteratively moved and turned until it almost perfectly fits onto the mirrored bone model.[8] Once the proximal bone models have been perfectly aligned, the deformity of the distal bone areas become visible. To verify the deformity in all 6° of freedom (3° of freedom for rotation and translation) the osteotomy is virtually simulated on the computer.[5]

The surgeon needs to determine the plane of osteotomy based on the former fracture line. The bone is then cut virtually, allowing free movement of the distal pathologic bone area, which is moved (by using the iterative closed point methodology) until fitting perfectly over the healthy side.[8] Sometimes, manual corrections or amendments are needed to achieve a perfectly planned clinical result.

Once the optimal correction has been achieved, an exact and computerized surgical plan is established using the CASPA software. This includes the accurate calculation of the plane(s) of osteotomy, the assessment of implants, and lastly the patient-specific guides for saws, drills, and reduction maneuvers. Those guides allow the proper translation from the virtually planned model into the true in vivo surgical result.[5]

In cases of closing-wedge osteotomies, the cut is automatically planned by the software, creating a gap.

In cases of rotatory malalignment without length discrepancy, a single-plane osteotomy can be created, avoiding the presence of any gap between the bone fragments. The correction is achieved through simple rotation and translation of the bony fragments along the plane of the osteotomy. For proper identification of the plane position, the authors recommend using an additional 3-D model of the implants (including screws), which can be laid over the simulation.

The patient guides are printed in a specific 3-D printer using biocompatible synthetic materials. Easy handling of those 3D-printers and the virtual-planning software technology combined with low costs are responsible for increasing interest in this technology.

The guides are integrated directly in the 3-D planning and developed using the CASPA software.

Any guide should perfectly fit onto the surface of the bone. The surgeon makes the appropriate exposure, while protecting soft tissues and neurovascular structures, so the guide can be inserted. The undersurface of the guide is shaped as a perfect negative of the bony surface. This is important to guarantee a perfect fit during surgery. The guide itself can individually be modified to provide the best handling during operation as possible.

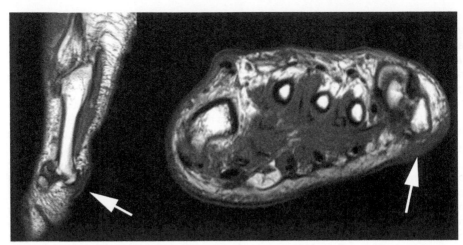

Fig. 1. The MRIs demonstrate the local ulceration under the left fifth MTP joint (*white arrows*). There is no sign of osteomyelitis or any other type of infection.

CASE EXAMPLE

This case illustrates the history of a 52-year-old, active woman who sustained minor foot trauma several years ago. Although she felt some pain over the area of the fourth and fifth toes, she never sought medical help. This led, due the coexisting malalignment of the fourth and fifth toes, to her developing ulcerations at the plantar aspect of the fifth metatarsophalangeal (MTP) joint (**Fig. 1**).

Conservative measures, including offloading insoles and adequate antibiotic treatment (applied by the family physician), reduced the ulceration to some extent. But, when the patient went back to regular life activity, the ulceration started to recur. This was the reason for her referral to the authors' clinic.

During the initial work-up, conventional radiographs were performed (**Fig. 2**) and revealed a malalignment of the fourth and fifth metatarsal bones after subcapital

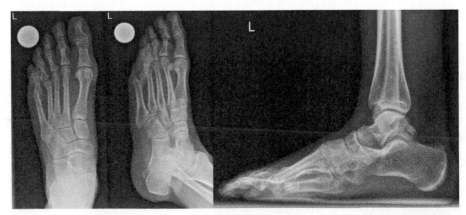

Fig. 2. Conventional radiographs of the left foot and ankle in 3 planes. Those were taken as part of the initial work-up. The images show a severe malalignment of the fourth and fifth metatarsal bones.

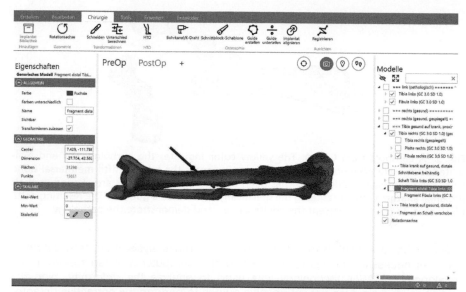

Fig. 3. Screenshots as obtained by the authors' developed software, CASPA. The tibia and fibula are seen. The pathologic side is of yellow color and the contralateral healthy (mirrored) side green. Alignment occurred by using the algorithm at the proximal anatomic structures to detect CORA and misalignment of the pathologic side. The software allows exact measurements of all necessary parameters to obtain the axis of corrective osteotomy.

fracture. As a consecutive sequela, a hammertoe deformity of the fourth and fifth toe resulted.

The MRI, in order to detect osteomyelitis, showed no signs of osteomyelitis within the head of the fifth metatarsal bone. Due to recurring ulcerations caused by significant misalignment of the fourth and fifth toe, surgical correction of the bony deformity has been discussed with the patient.

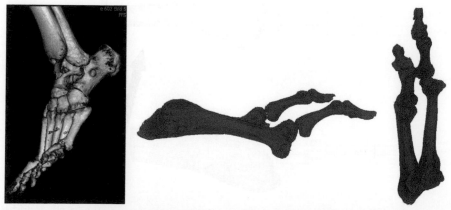

Fig. 4. (*Left*) The CT scan as performed using the special protocol for automated segmentation. (*Middle, Right*) The 3-D surface models obtained from the CT data are seen.

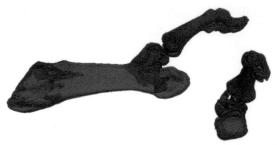

Fig. 5. Screenshots from CASPA. The yellow color indicates the pathologically and mal-united fifth metatarsal bone. The green color indicates the healthy fifth metatarsal bone from the contralateral side, which has been mirrored. The 2 models are aligned at their proximal anatomic structures using the specifically elaborated algorithm. The resulting delta pixels that do not fit, represent the "delta-value" and demonstrate the pathology.

Due to the severity of deformation, a more in-depth analysis of the bony deformation was necessary. In this case, the authors' computer-assisted research and development (CARD) technology was used to analyze the deformity, plan the correction, and produce patient-specific guides to perform the corrective osteotomies and guide the reduction of the fragments, according to the preoperative virtual planning.

STEP-BY-STEP PROCEDURE (TO EXPLAIN THE CORRECTION IN THE CASE)

The first step in the virtual planning is to obtain a 3-D model of the foot. To do so, CT data are needed. The CT scan is performed according to a particular protocol, and the generated data segmented using a special software (CASPA [**Fig. 3**]) to create editable models (**Fig. 4**).

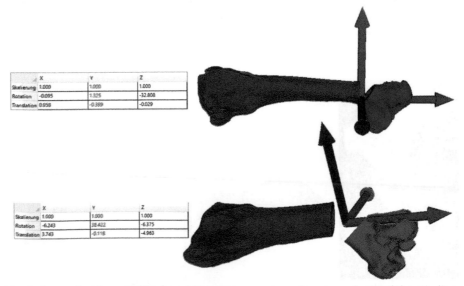

	X	Y	Z
Skalierung	1.000	1.000	1.000
Rotation	-0.095	1.325	-32.808
Translation	0.958	-0.389	-0.029

	X	Y	Z
Skalierung	1.000	1.000	1.000
Rotation	-6.243	38.422	-6.375
Translation	3.743	-0.118	-4.963

Fig. 6. Screenshot from CASPA for exact measurements, as done to understand the misalignment and to plan the correction.

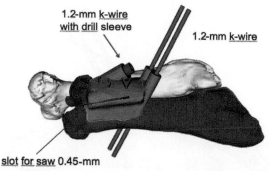

1.2-mm k-wire with drill sleeve

1.2-mm k-wire

slot for saw 0.45-mm

Fig. 7. Screenshot from CASPA. It shows the first step of the surgical technique in this particular case. The fifth metatarsal is shown with osteotomy guide mounted in place, which is held by 2 Kirschner (k-) wires. The purple object shows the removable drill sleeve for positioning of the third k-wire. In order to remove the osteotomy guide after performance of the first osteotomy the drill sleeve has to be removed. The k-wires have to stay in place.

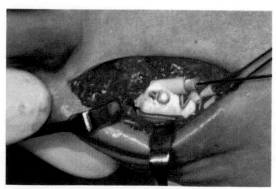

Fig. 8. Intraoperative photograph (the particular virtual planning image is shown in **Fig. 7**). Note the perfect fit of the osteotomy guide.

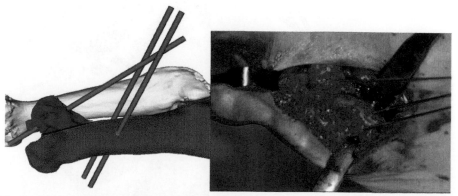

Fig. 9. Screenshot from CASPA and the corresponding intraoperative situs. The head fragment is cut and stabilized with the Kirschner wire in position. This Kirschner wire is used for the realignment guide after performing the second osteotomy.

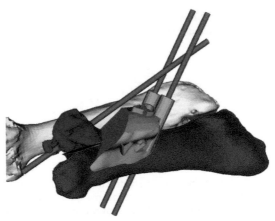

Fig. 10. Screenshot from CASPA showing the placement of the second osteotomy guide using the proximal Kirschner wires, which are left in place.

Using these data, a 3-D reconstruction of both the pathologic and healthy foot of the contralateral side can be done. The contralateral side is used as a template to help in the correction of the bone.

The healthy 3-D foot model is mirrored, and landmarks are registered over the area of most anatomic similarities (in this case, the proximal metatarsal bone area). After aligning the proximal region, the deformity is clearly (**Fig. 5**) visible.

By means of the software, the authors are able to simulate the osteotomies and the realignment to restore anatomy. After planning the corrective osteotomies and the realignment, the guides for surgical intervention and reduction are prepared. In the current case, the fragment is malunited, including an average dorsiflexion of 32°, and healed onto the metatarsal shaft (**Fig. 6**). To realign the bone, 2 osteotomies

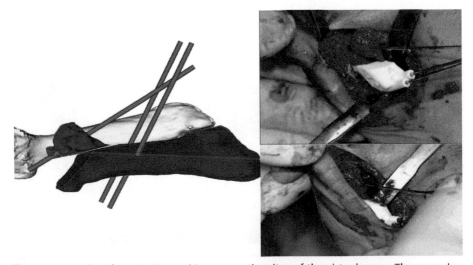

Fig. 11. Screenshot from CASPA and intraoperative situs of the virtual scene. The second osteotomy is performed to prepare the realignment of the head fragment.

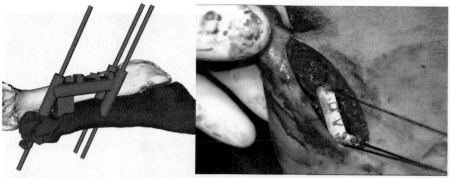

Fig. 12. Virtual planning image (*Left*) and its corresponding intraoperative photograph (*Right*). Screenshot from CASPA and intraoperative situs. The realignment guide is used to bring the head fragment in position. The visual control should show 3 parallel Kirschner wires.

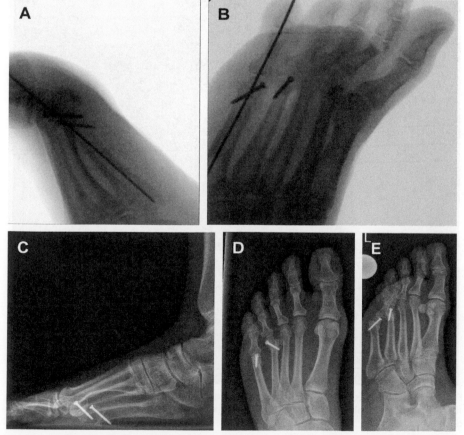

Fig. 13. (*A, B*) Intraoperative radiograph shows correct position of screws and Kirschner wire as correct position and alignment of fragments. One-year postintervention, patient is free from ulceration. (*C–E*) A slight dorsal deviation of the distal fragment of the fifth metarsal occurred without any clinical relevance. The alignment of fourth and fifth toes is still stable and no ulceration plantar has occurred.

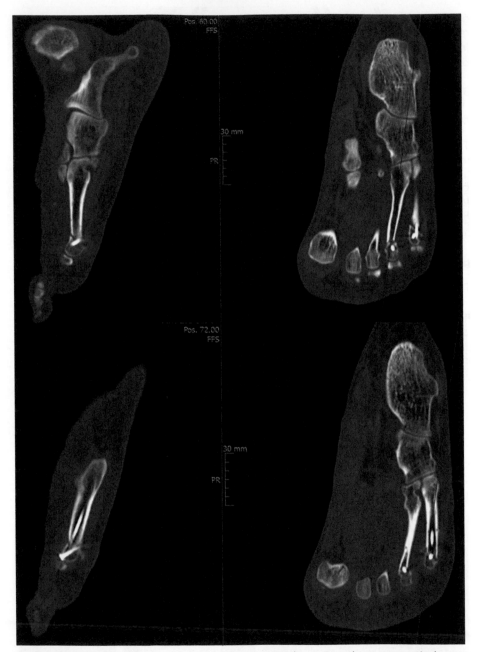

Fig. 14. Demonstrated are the CT scans of the presented case 6 weeks postoperatively, confirming anatomic realignment, as planned and executed using the software. Bony consolidation has begun.

are necessary. The first osteotomy is chosen horizontally to loosen the head fragment and to obtain the optimal level to realign the head fragment. The second osteotomy is to prepare the metatarsal shaft. The surgery (**Figs. 7–12**) is performed uneventfully. All guides fit perfectly onto the bone and reduction is achieved as planned. Intraoperative radiograph shows regular alignment and correct length and position of screws and fragments. A check-up 6 weeks postoperatively shows regular bone healing and stable correction (**Figs. 13** and **14**).

Any ulceration has been prevented and the patient has remained pain-free for 3 years.

SUMMARY

The use of specific software for virtual planning has shown effective for both major and minor complex deformity corrections. The greatest advantage is accurate preoperative planning, allowing simulation of the correction, to enable the best outcome. Once the perfect correction has been created virtually on a computer, it can be transferred to the operating room. By means of individually designed patient-specific guides, the whole surgical procedure can be performed safely and efficiently. This technique is an exciting development that will benefit from further research.

DISCLOSURE

The authors have nothing to disclose.

REFERENCES

1. Lamm BM, Paley D. Deformity correction planning for hindfoot, ankle, and lower limb. Clin Podiatr Med Srug 2004;21:305–26.
2. Meyer DC, Siebenrock KA, Schiele B, et al. A new methodology for the planning of single-cut corrective osteotomies of mal-aligned long bones. Clin Biomech (Bristol, Avon) 2005;20:223–7.
3. Nagy L, Jankauskas L, Dumont CE. Correction of forearm malunion guided by the preoperative complaint. Clin Orthop Relat Res 2008;466:1419–28.
4. Schweizer A, Fürnstahl P, Nagy L. Three-dimensional correction of distal radius intra-articula malunions using patient-specific-drill guides. J Hand Surg 2013; 38:2339–47.
5. Wirth SH, Espinosa N, Renner N, et al. Computer-aided three dimensional surgical planning with patient-specific instruments for accurate correction of mala-ligned bones of the foot and ankle. Fuss und Sprunggelenk 2015;13:123–32.
6. Mast JW, Teitge RA, Gowda M. Preoperative planning for the treatment of non-unions and the correction of malunions of the long bones. Orthop Clin North Am 1990;21:693–714.
7. Mast JW. Preoperative planning in the surgical correction of tibial nonunions and malunions. Clin Orthop Relat Res 1983;178:26–30.
8. Schweizer A, Fürnstahl P, Harders M, et al. Complex radius shaft malunion: ostoetomy with computer-assisted planning. Hand (NY) 2010;5:171–8.
9. Victor J, Premanthan A. Virtual 3D planning and patient specific surgical guides for ostoetomies around the knee: a feasibility and proof-of-concept study. Bone Joint J 2013;95B:153–8.
10. Lorensen WE, Cline HE. Marching cubes: a high resolution 3D surface construction algorithm. Comput Graph (ACM) 1987;21:163–9.
11. Ma B, Kunz M, Gammon B, et al. A laboratory comparison of computer navigation and individualized guides for distal radius osteotomies. Int J Comput Assist Radiol Surg 2014;9:713–24.

12. Miyake J, Murase T, Oka K, et al. Computer-assisted corrective osteotomy for malunited diaphyseal forearm fractures. J Bone Joint Surg Am 2012;94:150.
13. Athwal GS, Ellis RE, Small CF, et al. Computer-assisted distal radius osteotomy. J Hand Surg 2003;28:951–8.
14. Besl PJ, McKay ND. A method for registration of 3-D shapes. Pattern analysis and machine intelligence. IEEE Trans Med Imaging 1992;25(3):239–56.

Treatment of Stage 4 Flatfoot

Gavin Heyes, FRCS, MSc*, Andy Molloy, MBChB, MRCS, FRCS Tr&Orth

KEYWORDS

- Stage 4 flatfoot • Stage 4 posterior tibialis tendon dysfunction
- Stage 4 acquired adult flatfoot • Treatment • Surgical management

KEY POINTS

- Stage 4 flatfoot is rare, accounting for less than 3% of all flatfoot cases.
- Conservative treatment tends to only be successful in frail and low-demand patients.
- The greater the number of fused segments, the poorer the functional outcome.
- When considering joint-sparing surgery, hindfoot alignment must be neutral to reduce strain on the deltoid ligament complex and any subsequent reconstructions performed. Soft tissues must be balanced.

INTRODUCTION

Although flatfoot can have numerous causes, those caused by acquired deformity form the basis of the flatfoot classification[1,2] and discussion in this article. The medial longitudinal arch is a key structure during the gait cycle. Failure to maintain the alignment of the medial longitudinal arch has been shown to significantly affect gait, with cadence, stride length, speed, and stance all being significantly reduced. It has also been shown that, with increasing flatfoot severity, there is a decreasing range of motion in the ankle, hindfoot, and forefoot in all planes of motion. Overall, symptomatic flatfeet have worse kinematics in all modes of testing compared with asymptomatic feet.[3]

Alignment of the medial longitudinal arch is provided by its bony architecture, the plantar fascia, posterior tibial tendon (PTT), calcaneonavicular (spring) ligament, and naviculocuneiform ligament. One important element of the medial longitudinal arch is the orientation of the talonavicular joint. The spring ligament is a critical supporting structure, forming a sling within the acetabulum pedis. Recently the naviculocuneiform ligament has been identified as a separate structure to the PTT, important in stabilizing the naviculocuneiform joint and preventing a break in the Meary line at that joint.[4]

Department of Trauma and Orthopaedic Surgery, Aintree University Hospital, Lower Lane, Liverpool L9 7AL, UK
* Corresponding author.
E-mail address: gjheyes@live.co.uk

Foot Ankle Clin N Am 25 (2020) 269–280
https://doi.org/10.1016/j.fcl.2020.02.002
foot.theclinics.com

There are many reports of PTT dysfunction as the primary driver of flatfoot deformity.[5–9] However, more recently there has been increasing evidence that failure of the spring ligament alone is sufficient to cause flatfoot.[10,11] Whether the initial driver of the deformity is failure to the spring ligament or tibialis posterior, the end result is the same: a stage 4 flatfoot.

ORIGIN OF CLASSIFICATION

The clinical pattern now described as stage 4 flatfoot was initially suggested as a possible entity by Johnson and Strom[12] in 1989. It was reported as the end stage of a disorder initiated by PTT dysfunction. They described it as any case where, "the hindfoot has become fixed in eversion, over a number of years, to produce a valgus tilt of the talus within the ankle mortise and lateral tibiotalar degeneration." They also suggested that this pattern of deformity may be seen with or without prior history of trauma.[12] In 1997, the fourth stage of the classification was formalized by Myerson,[2] describing it as a rigid hindfoot, hindfoot malalignment as described in earlier stages, with valgus angulation of the talus and early degeneration of the ankle joint.[2] Stage 4 was subclassified as:

- Type 4a: those with a flexible ankle deformity amenable to ankle preservation with a deltoid reconstruction.
- Type 4b: those with fixed ankle deformities requiring a pantalar fusion.

The complete classification as described by Bluman and colleagues,[11] is shown in **Table 1**.

Both classifications were described for the sequelae of PTT dysfunction. As such, recommendations for treatment do not take into consideration all permeations of flatfoot deformity, which is perhaps why both classifications have not been validated in the literature.[13] It is imperative, in comparing treatments and outcomes, that like are compared with like; further studies are necessary to enable this.

Investigations

Radiographs

Standard radiographs include weight-bearing anteroposterior, oblique, and lateral views of foot and anteroposterior and lateral views of ankle. Radiographs of the contralateral side are useful for comparison when other causes of flatfoot are to be considered. Hindfoot alignment and long-leg views may also be required where there is uncertainty regarding the center of deformity.

Radiological parameters to be examined include, on the anteroposterior view, the talar first metatarsal angle and the talonavicular uncoverage angle. On the lateral view, parameters include the Meary line, calcaneal pitch, lateral tarsometatarsal angle, and medial cuneiform height.[14]

In stage 4 flatfoot, joint-preserving surgery in the foot is no longer possible. Radiographs facilitate identification of degenerate joints and also identify the location of the break in the radiological angles mentioned earlier.

MRI may help with confirmation of tibialis posterior, spring ligament, and deltoid ligament attenuation; however, in stage 4 flatfoot, that diagnosis can often be made through clinical examination and plain films. When joint-preserving surgery of the ankle is being considered, MRI may also facilitate the evaluation of residual cartilage because radiographs are not able to get the typical orthogonal views of the joints.

Table 1
Classification of posterior tibial tendon rupture

Stage	Substage	Most Characteristic Clinical Findings	Most Characteristic Radiographic Findings	Treatment
I	A	Normal anatomy Tenderness along PTT	Normal	Immobilization, NSAIDs, cryotherapy, orthoses, tenosynovectomy ± Systemic disease-specific pharmacotherapy
	B	Normal anatomy; tenderness along PTT	Normal	Immobilization, NSAIDs, cryotherapy, orthoses, tenosynovectomy
	C	Slight HF valgus; tenderness along PTT	Slight HF valgus	Immobilization, NSAIDs, cryotherapy, orthoses, tenosynovectomy
II	A1	Supple HF valgus Flexible forefoot varus Possible pain along PTT	HF valgus Meary line disruption Loss of calcaneal pitch	Orthoses Medial displacement calcaneal osteotomy TAL or Strayer and FDL transfer if deformity corrects only with ankle plantarflexion
	A2	Supple HF valgus Fixed forefoot varus Possible pain along PTT	HF valgus Meary line disruption Loss of calcaneal pitch	Orthoses Medial displacement calcaneal osteotomy and FDL transfer Cotton osteotomy
	B	Supple HF valgus Forefoot abduction	HF valgus Talonavicular uncovering Forefoot abduction	Orthoses Medial displacement calcaneal osteotomy and FDL transfer, lateral column lengthening
	C	Supple HF valgus Fixed forefoot varus Medial column instability First ray dorsiflexion with HF correction Sinus tarsi pain	HF valgus First TMT plantar gapping	Medial displacement calcaneal osteotomy and FDL transfer Cotton osteotomy or medial column fusion
III	A	Rigid HF valgus Pain in sinus tarsi	Subtalar joint space loss HF valgus Angle of Gissane sclerosis	Custom bracing if not surgical candidate Triple arthrodesis
	B	Rigid HF valgus Forefoot abduction Pain in sinus tarsi	Subtalar joint space loss HF valgus Angle of Gissane sclerosis Forefoot abduction	Custom bracing if not surgical candidate Triple arthrodesis ± lateral column lengthening
IV	A	Supple tibiotalar valgus	Tibiotalar valgus HF valgus	Surgery for HF valgus and associated deformity Deltoid reconstruction
	B	Rigid tibiotalar valgus	Tibiotalar valgus HF valgus	TTC fusion or pantalar fusion

Abbreviations: FDL, flexor digitorum longus; HF, hindfoot; NSAIDs, nonsteroidal antiinflammatory drugs; TAL, tendo achilles lengthening; TMT, tarsometatarsal joint; TTC, tibiotalocalcaneal.
From Bluman EM, Title CI, Myerson MS. Posterior tibial tendon rupture: a refined classification system. Foot Ankle Clin. 2007;12(2):233-49, v.; with permission.

Computed tomography (CT) scans are not routinely required for diagnostic purposes but can be of use in identifying the extent of degenerative change within the joints of the foot and quantify any bone loss.

TREATMENT

There is little in the way of evidence in the literature for nonoperative management of stage 4 flatfoot; however, in some patients, particularly the frail, a well-fitted orthosis can provide suitable pain relief to meet functional demands. Although numbers were low, 1 study reported reasonable results with a molded ankle foot orthosis (MAFO) in elderly patients with low functional demand. The caveat was that in those with poor balance or difficulty with ambulation (eg, Parkinson disease), their function deteriorated further with an MAFO.[7] Some success with a short hinged ankle foot orthosis (Marzano brace) has been noted in those with poor ambulation.[15] Regardless of the type of orthosis used, all function to accommodate deformity and, as such, do not correct tibiotalar valgus, which contributes to increased load going through the joint, progressive degenerative change, and poorer outcome in more active individuals.[1]

Traditionally, operative treatment of stage 4 flatfoot was in the form of a tibiotalocalcaneal (TTC) arthrodesis or pantalar arthrodesis. For flexible stage 4(a), more contemporary treatments include hindfoot realignment through limited arthrodeses and deltoid reconstruction. The level of evidence for all forms of treatment is low, which may in part be caused by the rarity of stage 4 disease.

Joint-preserving Surgery

For the purpose of this article, the joint to be preserved is the ankle joint, with the focus of the discussion revolving around its management. In general, this is reserved for cases of stage 4a flatfoot, where the joint is reducible, retains mobility, and retains most of its articular surface, or at least significant parts of the medial side. There is insufficient evidence in the literature regarding the best management approach for the hindfoot, whether that be a medial approach double, medial/dorsal and lateral approach double or triple arthrodesis. However, there is some evidence, and it is the authors' experience, that the medial approach significantly decreases wound complication rates because the incision is not under tension. In addition, the tendency while debriding a joint is to take more bone away from the side closest to the incision. A medial approach can therefore help in reducing the deformity.

Whatever approach is used, if a triple arthrodesis is left in residual hindfoot valgus, greater strain on deltoid ligament, attenuation of the deltoid ligament, and a residual valgus tibiotalar joint deformity have been reported.[16–18] It is therefore critical that anatomic alignment of the hindfoot is achieved to facilitate balancing of the ankle.

Fig. 1 shows typical stage 4 flatfoot radiographs. Note the negative Meary angle; in this instance the break is at the naviculocuneiform joint and there is a very low calcaneal pitch, significant hindfoot valgus, tibiotalar joint valgus, and marked talonavicular joint uncoverage. There is also significant instability of the naviculocuneiform joint caused by failure of the naviculocuneiform ligament. Failure to address this will therefore not fully correct the deformity.

Fig. 2 shows the postoperative radiographs of the patient in **Fig. 1** after a medial double fusion extended to involve the naviculocuneiform joint. Radiographs show improved calcaneal pitch angle, normalization of Meary line, improved talus first metatarsal angle, and reduction of hindfoot valgus. This outcome has led to an improvement in tibiotalar alignment.

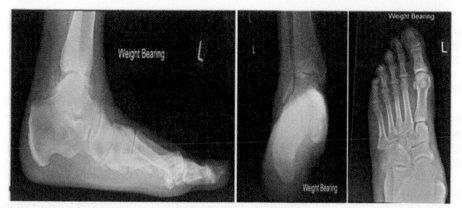

Fig. 1. Typical stage 4 flatfoot radiographs.

Once the hindfoot is balanced, the next thing to consider is soft tissue balancing of the ankle, and principally this involves addressing the deltoid ligament. Once again there is no strong evidence on how best to achieve this; often it is only mentioned broadly in review articles as a potential treatment modality. Deltoid ligament reconstructions have been reported using either tendon allograft[19,20] or local autograft from the peroneal longus,[21] flexor digitorum longus, or flexor hallucis longus tendon.[22]

Because of the infrequency of appropriate cases as well as the limited evidence to support its use, deltoid reconstructions in the presence of stage 4a flatfoot are very rarely performed at our institution. Our preference is to perform as a single procedure a hindfoot realignment and arthrodesis followed by reconstruction of the deltoid ligament anatomically where possible. This procedure is performed using a modification of the technique described by Myerson and colleagues[1]

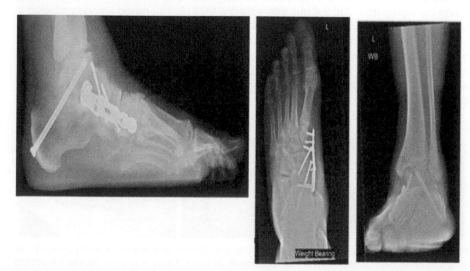

Fig. 2. Postoperative radiographs after medial double fusion extended to involve naviculo-cuneiform joint.

We use a hamstring allograft of at least 20 cm in length. It is thawed in warmed saline and whip stitches are placed on either end of tendon with 2 Vicryl. The middle of the graft is fixed using a tenodesis screw and blind bone tunnel at the origin of the deltoid on the medial malleolus (approximately at level of distal tibial physeal scar). The tendon is fixed distally with further blind bone tunnels and tenodesis screws at the level of the body of talus and sustenaculum tali.

Fig. 3A shows an extended medial approach to visualize the medial malleolus and origin of the deltoid ligament, **Fig. 3**B shows a subperiosteal flap developed at the deltoid origin and fixation of hamstring allograft, and **Fig. 3**C shows the orientation of the distal allograft toward the sustenaculum tali and the neck of the talus. Redundant deltoid ligament is plicated and used as an augment and double-breasted over-repair.

Postoperative management includes non–weight bearing in a cast for 6 weeks followed by a weight-bearing boot for a further 6 weeks.

With regard to results in the literature, 1 study reported outcomes of 8 patients with stage 4 flatfoot treated with hindfoot arthrodesis and deltoid ligament reconstruction using hamstring allograft and a minimally invasive approach.[20] Eight patients were followed up to 36 months. Radiological success was taken as a residual ankle valgus of less than 3°. At final follow-up, 5 patients (62.5%) maintained a successful radiological appearance. Patients in the successful and unsuccessful deltoid reconstruction groups were matched for age and body mass index. The 3 unsuccessful reconstructions went on to arthrodesis procedures. The magnitude of preoperative tibiotalar tilt is predictive of outcome, with recommendation that a joint-sparing procedure should be considered for tibiotalar angles of less than 10° valgus.[20]

Deland and colleagues[23] reported on the results of 5 patients that underwent deltoid ligament reconstruction using peroneal tendon autograft. Their cutoff for radiological success was a valgus tilt of 4° or less. At 2 years, they reported radiological success in 4 patients (80%). Functional outcomes were not reported in their initial results.

Long-term follow-up of the same group of patients to a mean of 8.9 years reported Foot and Ankle Outcome Score (FAOS) at final follow-up of 68.3 and Short-form 36 (SF-36) of 75.7. They were all able to walk between 10 and 40 blocks a day. Arthritis grade increased from 2 to 2.4 but, interestingly, they did not report any degradation in patient functional outcomes. Ankle range of motion ranged between 40° and 55° (dorsiflexion 0°–10°). Although outcomes are encouraging, it should be borne in mind that hindfoot was not fused and was addressed using calcaneal osteotomies and assorted forefoot procedures. There was limited discussion regarding graft site morbidity. In addition, FAOS scores are only validated for lateral ligament reconstruction outcomes.[21]

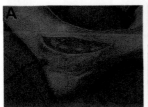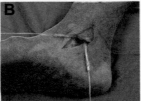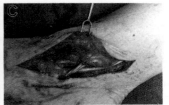

Fig. 3. (*A*) An extended medial approach to visualize the medial malleolus and origin of deltoid ligament. (*B*) A subperiosteal flap developed at deltoid origin and fixation of hamstring allograft. (*C*) The orientation of distal allograft toward sustenaculum tali and neck of talus. (*Courtesy of* M.S. Myerson, MD, Baltimore, MD.)

Their findings regarding the condition of the ankle joint are similar to those reported after long-term follow-up of patients after triple arthrodesis. Pell and colleagues[24] followed up 111 patients over a range of 2 to 10.8 years and reported that arthritis of the ankle was radiologically significantly more severe at end of follow-up. However, patient satisfaction was not associated with degree of arthritis. The main predictor of satisfaction was postoperative alignment. This represents the approach taken by the authors in addressing stage 4 flatfoot deformities in elderly patients who have the potential to be active. If there is valgus ankle arthritis that is not end stage, with most of the symptoms coming from the hindfoot, a correctly aligned triple arthrodesis plus or minus medial displacement, calcaneal osteotomy can help offload the symptomatic lateral part of the ankle joint and prevent the deltoid ligament from being stretched. Our experience is that this can provide better ambulation than a pantalar fusion, in these selected cases.

Tibiotalocalcaneal Arthrodesis

The main forms of joint-sacrificing surgery and fixation reported in the literature are either compression plating or through an intramedullary device. Screw-only fixation has fallen from favor and this is likely because of the significantly poorer compression and stability that has been proved in biomechanical studies.[25]

Tibiotalocalcaneal arthrodesis with intramedullary nail

The clinical picture of advanced flatfoot with degenerative change rarely presents with isolated arthritis in the ankle and subtalar joint and preservation of talonavicular and calcaneocuboid joints. As a result, outcomes in the literature are hard to come by. With regard to TTC arthrodesis, there are no published studies on outcomes for the treatment of stage 4 flatfoot. There are only published studies on TTC arthrodesis in degenerate hindfoot disorders of heterogeneous causes and patient groups. Some articles have combined results for intramedullary, screw and plate, and screw fixation.[26]

Almost all of the literature reports outcomes for open joint preparation. The authors typically perform this via a transfibular approach. An acetabular reamer is used to remove most of the required fibula, thus providing a good volume of graft. The joints are prepared retaining as much bone stock as possible with flexible chisels. An additional longitudinal incision is made in the medial gutter so that it may be prepared. This incision means that, on reducing the joint, the talus can be keyed into the medial corner of the plafond, being held by provisional wire fixation, which aids in reducing the deformity correctly (**Fig. 4**A). Any lateral defects are then filled with the autograft. Surgeons need to ensure that the heel is properly reduced and is then held with an intramedullary wire. If it is not properly reduced, then the entry point for the nail can be too medial on the calcaneus, even "blowing out" the medial wall or providing insufficient fix. Patients are treated non–weight bearing in a backslab until the wounds are healed. Weight bearing can then be commenced in a boot until union is confirmed (**Fig. 4**B).

Surgeons using retrograde intramedullary nailing as their chosen method of fixation report union rates of 75% to 92%.[27–32] There was a general trend for smaller, and likely underpowered, studies to report higher union rates.[29] It is also worth noting that 1 meta-analysis extracted 85 nonunions from articles in the literature and noted that only 26% required or opted for revision surgery.[29] This finding highlights an additional benefit of the intramedullary nail to provide adequate stability, even in nonunions, to allow patients to manage their symptoms. There is emerging evidence that sustained dynamic compression nails may reduce the time to union compared with conventional intramedullary nailing systems.[32]

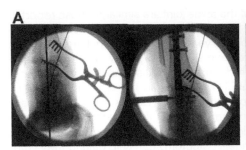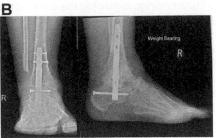

Fig. 4. (A) Fluoroscopic images showing reduction of the prepared joints with the talus keyed into the medial corner of plafond. (B) Postoperative radiographs after transfibular approach, reduction of the hindfoot, and fusion of both the tibiotalar and subtalar joint with an intramedullary nail.

In 1 article using a pain scale of 0 to 10, the mean pain score was 2 after completed follow-up.[27] SF-36 scores after completed follow-up showed improved physical function and mental health, but none achieved near-normal scores, highlighting that patients should expect some loss of function and pain compared with normal. However, 1 multicenter national study reported that all those that could not work because of their symptoms were able to return to work after TTC arthrodesis.[27,30,31]

Overall complication rates are reported at up to 24% to 55%.[27–29,33,34] Complications include malunion rates of up to 8% (typically increased hindfoot valgus), metalwork failure of up to 5%, and a combined superficial and deep infection rate of between 5% and 9%, Amputation rates were reported at 2% to 4.7%[29] and the iatrogenic perioperative fracture and tibial stress fracture rate was up to 5% to 18%.[27,28,33] Methods of reducing risk of fracture have been reported to include use of dynamic locking, nails with an in-built valgus, and longer nails.[29,35] The type of nail was often not clearly described in the literature.

Tibiotalocalcaneal Arthrodesis with Lateral Compression Plate

There is a paucity of data on plate fixation in the literature compared with intramedullary fixation. With regard to surgical approach for joint preparation and plate fixation, a lateral transfibular approach is favored in the literature.[36,37] This approach is preferred because it provides through a single wound adequate exposure to both joints, access to bone graft, an approach in between vascular pedicles, and good soft tissue coverage of metalwork, minimizing metalwork prominence. It is also a useful approach for a tension-free exposure. Compression is achieved across the joint with cannulated screws with an additional placement of the lateral plate, which provides additional compression as well as neutralization of potential deforming forces (**Fig. 5**). Our postoperative approach for this method of fixation is the same as for an intramedullary nail.

Results in the literature are similar to intramedullary nail fixation with significant improvement in functional scores, improvement in American Orthopaedic Foot and Ankle Society (AOFAS) score from 41 to 63, and reduction in pain scores from 7 to 3.[36] The union rate in 1 study was 12 of 13 patients.[36] Another article reported 100% union rate, in 12 patients, with cannulated screw and reverse Philos fixation through a transfibular approach.[37]

The investigators confirmed union by CT, and their postoperative mean AOFAS score was 77.5. They had no wound necrosis or infection but did have 1 case of lateral foot numbness.[37]

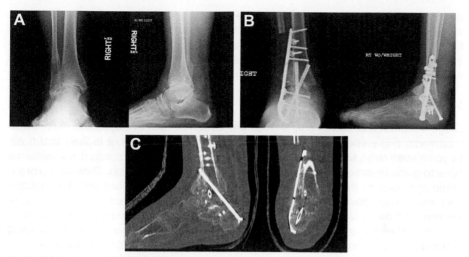

Fig. 5. (*A*) Preoperative radiographs of severe stage 4 flatfoot with stress fracture. (*B*) Postoperative radiographs of transfibular approach TTC with a lateral compression plate. (*C*) CT scans confirming union. ([*A, B*] *Courtesy of* M.S. Myerson, MD, Baltimore, MD.)

Pantalar Arthrodesis

There is no significant evidence in the literature on pantalar arthrodesis for stage 4 flatfoot. One study by Papa and colleagues[38] compared 8 pantalar arthrodeses and 13 TTC arthrodeses for posttraumatic arthritis. It was unclear in this study whether any of the cases also had a fixed flatfoot deformity. Overall, an 86% union rate was achieved, and there was a 10% wound complication rate and a 24% malunion rate. Patients with a TTC arthrodesis reported significantly better mobility and function compared with those that underwent a pantalar arthrodesis. Overall, of the 17 patients that were in employment before surgery, only 11 returned to work. The presence of diabetes and, in particular, neuropathy increases the risk of complications considerably, with a complication rate of 50% reported in an article by Herscovici and colleagues.[39] Both articles highlight that a pantalar arthrodesis is a technically challenging procedure that has risks and is likely to affect function. Given the impact of pantalar arthrodeses on function and stiffness, strong consideration should be given to joint-preserving surgery if possible.

Total ankle replacement

There is little in the literature regarding total ankle replacements in the setting of stage 4 flatfoot. One review article has highlighted that their own institutional practice is that, in some select cases of stage 4b flatfoot, an ankle replacement may be considered. Their criteria were that the patient must be more than 60 years of age, have good neurovascular status, have no diabetes, and have ankle valgus of less than 15°.[5] On review of the literature, the authors could find no long-term data from that institution on outcomes.

One other article describing how to plan and manage total ankle replacements with flatfoot recommended a 2-stage procedure 3 months apart, with the first stage involving correction of hindfoot alignment through arthrodesis. During the second stage, an Agility total ankle replacement was performed with initial cuts with an external ankle distractor on, and, once at trial stage, any residual tilting was corrected through soft tissue releases (usually lateral structures). The importance of hindfoot alignment was highlighted. Should there be any residual hindfoot valgus following first stage of the procedure, then a medial displacement calcaneal osteotomy is performed. That article reported a 15% reoperation rate at 1 year. It noted component tilting on ambulation and subsidence as some of the main problems. The final outcomes were not reported.[40]

SUMMARY

Stage 4 flatfoot represents only a small proportion of flatfoot cases and, with better treatments and earlier interventions for lesser stages of flatfoot, it is likely that it will become even rarer. Much like other uncommon foot and ankle disorders, the evidence base to guide treatment is limited to case series and expert opinion. Therefore, a pragmatic approach to treatment must be taken. Low-demand individuals may manage well with conservative treatment. Surgical management is complex, likely to require staging, and has a significant complication profile. Patients should be fully informed and understanding of this. First principles of surgery should be followed, including restoring hindfoot and ankle joint alignment, appropriate soft tissue balancing, and optimizing function by limiting arthrodeses and subsequent stiffness where possible.

ACKNOWLEDGMENTS

The authors would like to thank Dr Mark Myerson for allowing them to use some of his clinical cases.

DISCLOSURE

The authors have nothing to disclose.

REFERENCES

1. Bluman EM, Myerson MS. Stage IV posterior tibial tendon rupture. Foot Ankle Clin 2007;12(2):341–62, viii.
2. Myerson MS. Adult acquired flatfoot deformity: treatment of dysfunction of the posterior tibial tendon. Instr Course Lect 1997;46:393–405.
3. Shin HS, Lee JH, Kim EJ, et al. Flatfoot deformity affected the kinematics of the foot and ankle in proportion to the severity of deformity. Gait Posture 2019;72: 123–8.
4. Swanton E, Fisher L, Fisher A, et al. An anatomic study of the naviculocuneiform ligament and its possible role maintaining the medial longitudinal arch. Foot Ankle Int 2019;40(3):352–5.
5. Vulcano E, Deland JT, Ellis SJ. Approach and treatment of the adult acquired flatfoot deformity. Curr Rev Musculoskelet Med 2013;6(4):294–303.
6. Ruffilli A, Traina F, Giannini S, et al. Surgical treatment of stage II posterior tibialis tendon dysfunction: ten-year clinical and radiographic results. Eur J Orthop Surg Traumatol 2018;28(1):139–45.
7. Chao W, Wapner KL, Lee TH, et al. Nonoperative management of posterior tibial tendon dysfunction. Foot Ankle Int 1996;17(12):736–41.
8. Deland JT, de Asla RJ, Sung IH, et al. Posterior tibial tendon insufficiency: which ligaments are involved? Foot Ankle Int 2005;26(6):427–35.
9. Goldner JL, Keats PK, Bassett FH 3rd, et al. Progressive talipes equinovalgus due to trauma or degeneration of the posterior tibial tendon and medial plantar ligaments. Orthop Clin North Am 1974;5(1):39–51.

10. Tryfonidis M, Jackson W, Mansour R, et al. Acquired adult flat foot due to isolated plantar calcaneonavicular (spring) ligament insufficiency with a normal tibialis posterior tendon. Foot Ankle Surg 2008;14(2):89–95.

11. Bluman EM, Title CI, Myerson MS. Posterior tibial tendon rupture: a refined classification system. Foot Ankle Clin 2007;12(2):233–49, v.

12. Johnson KA, Strom DE. Tibialis posterior tendon dysfunction. Clin Orthop Relat Res 1989;(239):196–206.

13. Abousayed MM, Tartaglione JP, Rosenbaum AJ, et al. Classifications in brief: johnson and strom classification of adult-acquired flatfoot deformity. Clin Orthop Relat Res 2016;474(2):588–93.

14. Soliman SB, Spicer PJ, van Holsbeeck MT. Sonographic and radiographic findings of posterior tibial tendon dysfunction: a practical step forward. Skeletal Radiol 2019;48(1):11–27.

15. Wapner KL, Chao W. Nonoperative treatment of posterior tibial tendon dysfunction. Clin Orthop Relat Res 1999;(365):39–45.

16. Kelly IP, Nunley JA. Treatment of stage 4 adult acquired flatfoot. Foot Ankle Clin 2001;6(1):167–78.

17. Song SJ, Lee S, O'Malley MJ, et al. Deltoid ligament strain after correction of acquired flatfoot deformity by triple arthrodesis. Foot Ankle Int 2000;21(7):573–7.

18. Resnick RB, Jahss MH, Choueka J, et al. Deltoid ligament forces after tibialis posterior tendon rupture: effects of triple arthrodesis and calcaneal displacement osteotomies. Foot Ankle Int 1995;16(1):14–20.

19. Kitaoka HB, Luo ZP, An KN. Reconstruction operations for acquired flatfoot: biomechanical evaluation. Foot Ankle Int 1998;19(4):203–7.

20. Jeng CL, Bluman EM, Myerson MS. Minimally invasive deltoid ligament reconstruction for stage IV flatfoot deformity. Foot Ankle Int 2011;32(1):21–30.

21. Ellis SJ, Williams BR, Wagshul AD, et al. Deltoid ligament reconstruction with peroneus longus autograft in flatfoot deformity. Foot Ankle Int 2010;31(9):781–9.

22. Bohay DR, Anderson JG. Stage IV posterior tibial tendon insufficiency: the tilted ankle. Foot Ankle Clin 2003;8(3):619–36.

23. Deland JT, de Asla RJ, Segal A. Reconstruction of the chronically failed deltoid ligament: a new technique. Foot Ankle Int 2004;25(11):795–9.

24. Pell RFT, Myerson MS, Schon LC. Clinical outcome after primary triple arthrodesis. J Bone Joint Surg Am 2000;82(1):47–57.

25. Hamid KS, Glisson RR, Morash JG, et al. Simultaneous intraoperative measurement of cadaver ankle and subtalar joint compression during arthrodesis with intramedullary nail, screws, and tibiotalocalcaneal plate. Foot Ankle Int 2018;39(9):1128–32.

26. Chou LB, Mann RA, Yaszay B, et al. Tibiotalocalcaneal arthrodesis. Foot Ankle Int 2000;21(10):804–8.

27. Rammelt S, Pyrc J, Agren PH, et al. Tibiotalocalcaneal fusion using the hindfoot arthrodesis nail: a multicenter study. Foot Ankle Int 2013;34(9):1245–55.

28. Pellegrini MJ, Schiff AP, Adams SB Jr, et al. Outcomes of tibiotalocalcaneal arthrodesis through a posterior achilles tendon-splitting approach. Foot Ankle Int 2016;37(3):312–9.

29. Jehan S, Shakeel M, Bing AJ, et al. The success of tibiotalocalcaneal arthrodesis with intramedullary nailing–a systematic review of the literature. Acta Orthop Belg 2011;77(5):644–51.

30. Millett PJ, O'Malley MJ, Tolo ET, et al. Tibiotalocalcaneal fusion with a retrograde intramedullary nail: clinical and functional outcomes. Am J Orthop (Belle Mead NJ) 2002;31(9):531–6.

31. Muckley T, Klos K, Drechsel T, et al. Short-term outcome of retrograde tibiotalocalcaneal arthrodesis with a curved intramedullary nail. Foot Ankle Int 2011; 32(1):47–56.
32. Steele JR, Kildow BJ, Cunningham DJ, et al. Comparison of tibiotalocalcaneal arthrodeses using a sustained dynamic compression nail versus nondynamized nails. Foot Ankle Spec 2019. https://doi.org/10.1177/1938640019843332.
33. Kile TA, Donnelly RE, Gehrke JC, et al. Tibiotalocalcaneal arthrodesis with an intramedullary device. Foot Ankle Int 1994;15(12):669–73.
34. Lucas YHJ, Abad J, Remy S, et al. Tibiotalocalcaneal arthrodesis using a straight intramedullary nail. Foot Ankle Int 2015;36(5):539–46.
35. Dominic Marley W, Tucker A, McKenna S, et al. Pre-requisites for optimum centering of a tibiotalocalcaneal arthrodesis nail. Foot Ankle Surg 2014;20(3): 215–20.
36. Coughlin MJ, Nery C, Baumfeld D, et al. Tibiotalocalcaneal arthrodesis with lateral compression plate: artrodese tibio-talo-calcaneana com placa de compressao lateral. Rev Bras Ortop 2012;47(4):467–73.
37. Fan J, Zhang X, Luo Y, et al. Tibiotalocalcaneal (TTC) arthrodesis with reverse PHILOS plate and medial cannulated screws with lateral approach. BMC Musculoskelet Disord 2017;18(1):317.
38. Papa JA, Myerson MS. Pantalar and tibiotalocalcaneal arthrodesis for post-traumatic osteoarthrosis of the ankle and hindfoot. J Bone Joint Surg Am 1992; 74(7):1042–9.
39. Herscovici D, Sammarco GJ, Sammarco VJ, et al. Pantalar arthrodesis for post-traumatic arthritis and diabetic neuroarthropathy of the ankle and hindfoot. Foot Ankle Int 2011;32(6):581–8.
40. Greisberg J, Hansen TS. Total ankle replacement in the advanced flatfoot. Tech Foot Ankle Surg 2003;2:152–61.

Salvage Arthrodesis for Failed Total Ankle Replacement

Samuel B. Adams, MD

KEYWORDS

- Failure • Ankle replacement • Ankle arthroplasty • Tibiotalar • Tibiotalocalcaneal
- 3D printing • Allograft

KEY POINTS

- Total ankle replacement failure continues to occur and there are limited choices for revision ankle replacement.
- Salvage arthrodesis for failed total ankle replacement can be a successful procedure with an initial overall fusion rate of 84%.
- However, the fusion results of tibiotalar arthrodesis are greater than tibiotalocalcaneal arthrodesis.
- In addition to the complexity of the arthrodesis, the choice of bone void filler and the presence of inflammatory joint disease can decrease the fusion rate.
- The following factors are the most important indications for salvage arthrodesis: severe loss of bone stock (tibia, talus, or both), inadequate soft tissue coverage, or the inability to eradicate an infection.

INTRODUCTION

Total ankle replacement (TAR) is a successful procedure for end-stage ankle arthritis with outcomes equivalent to ankle arthrodesis.[1] In fact, the use of TAR is steadily increasing[2]; likely secondary to an increasing number of reports documenting positive midterm results of multiple implants.[3–9] However, TAR may have more reoperations, revision procedures, and eventual failures compared with ankle arthrodesis.[1]

In an analysis of national registry data, Labek and colleagues[10] reported a primary TAR failure rate of 21.8% at 5 years and 43.5% after 10 years across multiple implants. As survival is expected to decrease with longer follow-up, risk factors for failure must be understood and reliable treatment options are needed. Risk factors for TAR failure are numerous and not completely known. For example, a recent study of 107 TARs reported that diabetes mellitus, a poor baseline Ankle Osteoarthritis Scale score, an

Division of Foot and Ankle Surgery, Department of Orthopaedic Surgery, Duke University Medical Center, 4709 Creekstone Drive, Durham, NC 27703, USA
E-mail address: Samuel.adams@duke.edu

Foot Ankle Clin N Am 25 (2020) 281–291
https://doi.org/10.1016/j.fcl.2020.02.003
1083-7515/20/© 2020 Elsevier Inc. All rights reserved.

foot.theclinics.com

excessively dorsiflexed talar component, and an anteriorly/posteriorly translated talus relative to the tibial axis were statistically associated with metal component failure.[11] However, another study of 533 ankles found only prosthesis type and ipsilateral hindfoot fusion as risk factors for failure.[12]

Successful revision TAR has been described. Ellington and colleagues[13] reported satisfactory postoperative patient reported outcomes on 41 revision TARs at a mean follow-up of 49.1 months. However, revision TAR is not always appropriate. In fact, the previously described study reported a 13% revision TAR failure rate leading to subsequent arthrodesis or amputation procedures. Revision arthroplasty is often impossible owing to severe loss of tibia or talus bone stock, soft tissue problems, or infection. In these scenarios, treatment guidelines are not well described. However, salvage tibiotalar (TT) or tibiotalocalcaneal (TTC) arthrodesis, and amputation are all viable options. Amputation is generally reserved for severe cases. This article focuses on the indications, treatment decision making, techniques, and outcomes of salvage arthrodesis for failed TAR.

INDICATIONS AND TREATMENT DECISION MAKING

The decision to perform salvage arthrodesis is based on many factors, but the following are the most important indications: severe loss of bone stock (tibia, talus, or both), inadequate soft tissue coverage, or the inability to eradicate an infection. With few revision implants on the market, salvage arthrodesis is currently the most common treatment for failed TAR and justification for revision TAR is limited when any of these factors are present.

Many approaches to achieve stable TT or TTC fusion after TAR failure have been described. Published techniques include the use of plates and screws when adequate bone stock is available or, when there is inadequate bone stock, the use of retrograde intramedullary nails with or without structural bone graft, prefabricated metal implants, or custom 3-dimensional (3D)-printed implants. Circular external fixation has also been described in the setting of infection or acute shortening and proximal bone transport for inadequate bone stock. However, there is no comparison literature to guide treatment decisions in salvage arthrodesis; therefore, the choice of technique can be difficult. We discuss the author's general algorithm for salvage arthrodesis (**Fig. 1**).

Tibiotalar Versus Tibiotalocalcaneal Arthrodesis

Whenever possible, TT arthrodesis should be performed over TTC arthrodesis. Intuitively, TT arthrodesis is favorable to preserve subtalar and hindfoot motion. However, function after TT and TTC has rarely been compared. Although not in the setting of salvage arthrodesis, Ajis and colleagues[14] demonstrated no significant difference in patient satisfaction and return to activity when comparing TT and TTC arthrodesis. However, often a TTC arthrodesis must be performed because of (1) limited talus bone stock for adequate fixation, (2) subtalar arthritis, and (3) damage to the subtalar joint by subsided talus component.

Of these 3 scenarios, limited talus bone stock is the most subjective for determining if TT arthrodesis is appropriate. Kruidenier and colleagues,[15] in a series of TT and TTC arthrodesis, chose intramedullary nailing and TTC arthrodesis when significant bone loss was present, but there are no criteria for determining a critical amount of bone loss. The key determinants for adequate talus bone stock are (1) can stable fixation be achieved and (2) can osseous healing occur across the interfaces. The most commonly used fixation method for TT arthrodesis is anterior plating. The author prefers this method (**Fig. 2B**). However, for any method, stable fixation in the talar neck

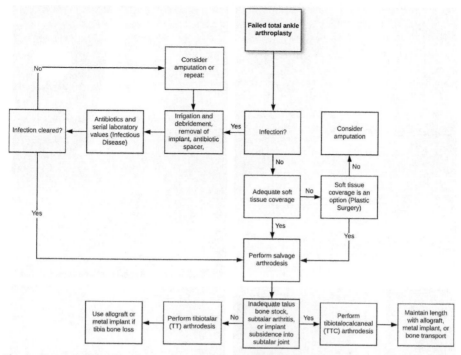

Fig. 1. General algorithm for performing salvage arthrodesis after failed TAR.

and preferably the talar body must be achieved. This goal is nearly impossible when the bone stock of the talus falls below the level of the navicular in the sagittal plane. Moreover, with little talus bone left, the body's ability to mount a bone healing response is limited. Therefore, when the bone stock falls below the level of the navicular in the sagittal plane, TTC arthrodesis should be considered over TT arthrodesis (**Fig. 2**).

Addressing Limited Bone Stock

There are several ways to address limited bone stock. These include autograft, allograft (typically femoral head), a noncustom metal cage, and a custom 3D-printed metal cage. However, there are no comparison studies to help guide the treating surgeon. In general, an autograft is not sufficient in size and structural support to address the bone void after failed TAR. The most common graft method for filling bone voids around the ankle is a bulk femoral head allograft. Although not all cases were for failed TAR, Jeng and colleagues[16] reported on the use of bulk femoral head allograft to treat bone defects of the ankle in 32 patients. They reported a 50% fusion rate, although nonunions were largely driven by diabetic patients. They also reported significant graft collapse in the nonunion group.

In an attempt to increase the union rate and avoid graft collapse, metal implants have been used to span large bone defects about the ankle, but the data are limited. A small series of 3 patients who received a trabecular metal implant for TT or TTC salvage arthrodesis demonstrated radiographic (non-computed tomography) healing and satisfactory outcomes at a mean of 57 months after surgery.[17] However, Aubret and colleagues[18] recently reported continued pain and difficulty assessing arthrodesis

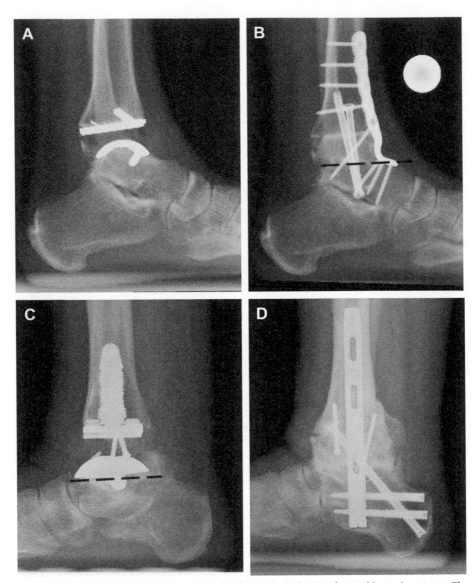

Fig. 2. (*A*) Lateral radiograph of a patient with continued pain after ankle replacement. The patient was found to have aseptic loosening at the time of surgery. He opted for a TT arthrodesis instead of a revision ankle replacement. (*B*) Lateral radiograph after TT fusion. The dotted line represents the talus height (after of removal of implants and debridement). The dotted line is dorsal to the navicular, which is a good reference point to determine if there is adequate bone stock for a TT arthrodesis. (*C*) Lateral radiograph of a failed TAR. The talar component has collapsed below the level of the navicular (*dotted line*), indicated inadequate bone stock for TT arthrodesis. (*D*) Lateral radiograph of the same patient from *C* after TTC arthrodesis.

in a series of patients who received trabecular metal implants for failed TAR. This author recently reported on 15 patients who received a custom 3D cage for large bone defects about the ankle.[19] There were 2 failures, one for nonunion and one for infection. There are no data to support one of these methods over the other.

Currently, this author prefers to use either a spherical femoral head or a spherical 3D implant (**Fig. 3**). The use of spherical graft/implant provides substantial bony contact and the freedom for infinite foot positioning. The foot can be rotated around the spherical implant to achieve the desired position. After implant removal and initial debridement of the bone surfaces, an acetabular reamer, approximately corresponding with the size of the femoral head or implant, is used to create a spherical cavity of bleeding bone surface out of the distal tibia, talus, and navicular. If the talus is deficient, the acetabular reamer can also be used to create a concave surface out of the posterior facet of the calcaneus. Typically, the femoral head is decorticated and injected with concentrated bone marrow aspirate. If using a 3D implant, it is packed with morcellized autograft fibula or a stem cell allograft (**Fig. 4**).

Infection

Not all TAR infections need to be treated with salvage arthrodesis.[20,21] However, infection is undoubtedly the most complicated scenario in salvage of failed TAR, because options to fill the void left by the TAR are even more problematic and fusion is difficult to achieve when infection is present. Allograft bone and metal cages are not appropriate in active infection. If salvage arthrodesis is the ultimate goal, over chronic cement spacer implantation or amputation, then appropriate practices should be used for infection eradication treatment. Consultation with an infectious disease physician should be performed. After appropriate antibiotics and an antibiotic holiday, the patient should undergo a repeat bone biopsy with culture to determine infection status. Salvage arthrodesis should not be performed until normalization of infection laboratory values and negative bone cultures. If infection is still present then 2 options exist: (1) an antibiotic-impregnated spacer with continued antibiotics and further debridements or (2) continued antibiotics with limb-shortening arthrodesis using a circular external fixation can be performed.

Inadequate Soft Tissue Coverage

Wound complications after total ankle arthroplasty range from 6.6% to 28% of patients.[22,23] Inadequate soft tissues are a problem for both revision TAR and salvage arthrodesis. In cases of inadequate soft tissue coverage, a plastic surgeon should be consulted to assess soft tissue coverage options and guide treatment. If options do not exist, consideration should be given to a below-the-knee amputation. If options

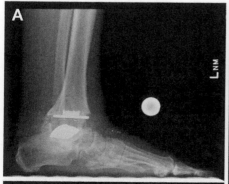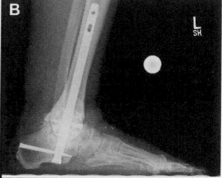

Fig. 3. (*A*) Lateral radiograph of a failed TAR with loss of bone stock, implant collapse into the subtalar joint, and subtalar joint arthritis. (*B*) Lateral radiograph after a custom 3D-printed spherical implant was used to perform a TTC arthrodesis. The patient is now pain free.

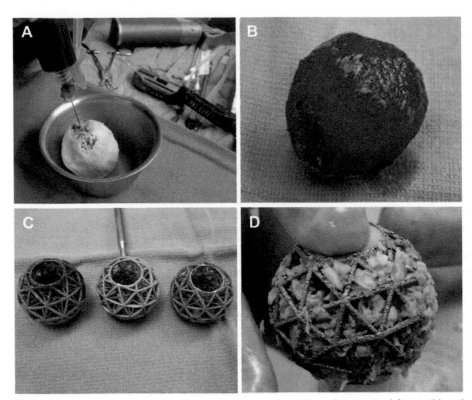

Fig. 4. (*A*) Concentrated bone marrow aspirate injection into a decorticated femoral head. (*B*) Decorticated femoral head is now completely filled with the patient's own concentrated bone marrow aspirate. (*C*) Three different sizes of a custom 3D-printed sphere. (*D*) The sphere has been packed with the patient's own morcellized fibula.

do exist, then salvage arthrodesis can be performed. Typically, the author performs the salvage arthrodesis in the same operative event as the soft tissue coverage procedure. Staged management of arthrodesis before coverage could allow for infection. In contrast, coverage before arthrodesis typically requires a waiting period of flap maturation and additional plastic surgery coordination before salvage arthrodesis.

OUTCOMES

Understanding the outcomes of salvage arthrodesis can be difficult. The literature is sparse and the titles of most articles include the words ankle arthrodesis but combine both TT and TTC arthrodeses in the results. Whenever possible, the results discussed herein are divided into TT and TTC arthrodesis. Moreover, fusion rates are reported, but the criteria for clinical and radiographic fusion differ among the studies, making comparisons difficult. In an attempt to synthesize these data, Gross and colleagues[24] performed a systematic review on salvage arthrodeses. The overall first attempt fusion rate of TT and TTC arthrodeses was 84%. However, when looking at TT and TTC arthrodeses separately, TT arthrodesis had a significantly higher first attempt fusion rate of 94% compared with 65% for TTC cases. However, the TTC arthrodeses were undertaken in cases where there was more significant bone loss, thereby making achievement of union more challenging.

When making the decision to perform primary TAR or TT arthrodesis on a patient with ankle arthritis, it is much too easy to recommend TAR and tell the patient that, if it fails, a TT arthrodesis can be performed. However, the outcomes of salvage TT and TTC arthrodesis are not as good as primary arthrodesis. In a matched pair study of both TT and TTC arthrodesis, Rahm and colleagues[25] demonstrated inferior clinical results with salvage arthrodesis compared with primary arthrodesis. Patients who underwent salvage arthrodesis showed significantly worse outcomes regarding the total Short Form-36, Short Form-36 physical function and Foot Function Index-D scores for pain and function. Primary arthrodesis patients had less pain and better function as well as improved quality of life when compared with salvage arthrodesis patients. Surprisingly, the union rates of salvage and primary arthrodeses were similar.

The largest study on failed TAR reported on 118 salvage arthrodeses.[26] The exact numbers of TT versus TTC arthrodeses were not reported, but the majority of these cases were performed with a retrograde TTC nail, indicating a TTC arthrodesis. The overall first attempt successful fusion rate was 90%. The most interesting data from this study regarded the patient reported outcomes measures that were given to a limited number of patients. The authors compared the outcomes of salvage arthrodesis in 10 of these patients with 7 patients who underwent revision TAR. The authors concluded that postoperative pain and the reoperation rate was higher in the revision TAR group and recommended salvage arthrodesis over revision for failed TAR. Deleu and colleagues[27] reported on 17 patients who underwent TT (5 patients) or TTC (12 patients) salvage arthrodesis. Thirteen patients (76%) achieved radiographic fusion on the first attempt. Not surprising, all 4 patients who did not achieve initial fusion underwent TTC arthrodesis. Of the 4 nonunions, 3 healed after a second attempt and 1 patient did not have a second attempt because the nonunion was asymptomatic.

When early aseptic loosening without talus bone collapse is encountered and revision TAR is not chosen as a treatment option, salvage arthrodesis without a graft is an option. Ali and colleagues[28] reported on 23 TTC arthrodeses for aseptic loosening of TARs. They used a retrograde hindfoot TTC intramedullary nail without any interpositional spacer or graft. The union rate for the ankle was 95% and the union rate for the subtalar joint was 91%. However, most often, resection of the ankle components leaves a large bone void. One study reported on the use of fresh frozen femoral heads for TTC salvage arthrodesis in 5 patients.[29] Despite the low number of patients, this study benefits the literature by reporting an average of 5-year results. In this group, 3 of 5 patients (60%) demonstrated complete healing of the graft. The nonunions occurred in 1 patient who had complete collapse of the graft and 1 patient who had a subtalar nonunion. In this series, the average limb length discrepancy at most recent follow-up was 1.6 cm, but 2 patients had discrepancies that were greater than 2 cm. This article highlights potential problems with the use femoral head allograft.

Alternatives to the use of femoral heads for filling bone voids in salvage TT or TTC arthrodeses include acute shortening with proximal bone transport, the use of so-called off-the-shelf metal implants, and custom 3D-printed implants. A recent study reported on poor outcomes with the use of a trabecular metal implant.[18] Eleven patients underwent either TTC (10 patients) or TT (1 patient) salvage arthrodesis with a trabecular metal ankle interpositional spacer. Patients were followed for a mean of 19 months and a minimum of 1 year. A computed tomography scan analysis of the fusion rate was difficult secondary to artifact from the metal implants. Fusion at the tibia–implant interface was more common than at the implant–calcaneus interface. Patients continued to complain of pain and had a most recent follow-up average American Orthopaedic Foot and Ankle Society score of 52 out of 100. The author recently reported on the use of custom 3D-printed cages for ankle and hindfoot arthrodeses.[19] Two of the 15 patients in this study underwent salvage TTC arthrodesis for failed TAR. Both successfully fused and were pain free (**Fig. 5**).

In an effort to combat limb length discrepancy, 1 study reported on the use of circular external fixation for salvage arthrodesis in 7 patients.[30] Four patients underwent TT arthrodesis and 3 patients underwent tibiocalcaneal arthrodesis. The mean bone stock deficit after TAR explantation was 5.1 cm (range, 3.7–8.5 cm). Moreover, 4 patients elected to have a lengthening procedure and 3 patients elected to use shoe lifts. Patients spent an average of 197 days (range, 149–229 days) in the circular external fixator. All patients achieved a solid fusion.

TAR has been recognized as a treatment option for rheumatoid arthritis, but the presence of the disease negatively influences implant survival. Because rheumatoid arthritis and rheumatoid arthritis treatment medicines are known to decrease bone healing, concern for union after salvage arthrodesis must be appreciated. One study compared fusion rates in patient with and without inflammatory joint disease.[15] The authors found a significantly higher fusion rate in patients without inflammatory joint disease (96% vs 73%). Similar results were obtained by Doets and Zurcher[31] Salvage arthrodesis was performed on 18 ankles. TT arthrodesis was performed on 7 patients and TTC arthrodesis was performed on 11 patients. Eleven of the 18 arthrodeses (61%) obtained fusion on the first attempt. All nonunions occurred in inflammatory joint disease patients.

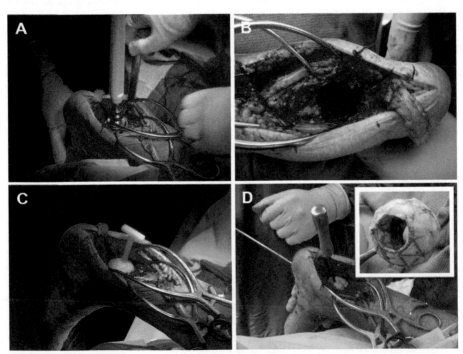

Fig. 5. (*A*) Intraoperative image of the use of an acetabular reamer to prepare the tibia and calcaneus after failed TAR. A posterior approach was used because of prior anterior wound healing problems. The TAR components were removed from this approach. (*B*) Spherical void left after reaming. (*C*) A 3D-printed trial inserted to ensure appropriate size. The trial is cannulated and reaming for intramedullary TTC nail placement was performed with the trial in place. (*D*) The 3D printed spherical implant was packed with bone graft and inserted.

A summary of these results indicates that salvage TT arthrodesis has a higher rate of first-time fusion than salvage TTC arthrodesis. Moreover, TT or TTC salvage arthrodesis is less satisfactory to patients compared with these same primary arthrodeses. A higher fusion rate can be expected with native bone is able to be used instead of an interpositional graft. Interpositional bone grafts can be subject to nonunion and collapse. The results of metal implants are not yet well defined. Inflammatory joint disease decreases the fusion rate of salvage arthrodesis.

SUMMARY

Salvage arthrodesis is a reliable treatment option for failed TAR. The decision to perform salvage arthrodesis is based on many factors including severe loss of bone stock (tibia, talus, or both), inadequate soft tissue coverage, or the inability to eradicate an infection. With few revision implants on the market, salvage arthrodesis is currently the most common treatment for failed TAR and justification for revision TAR is limited when any of these factors are present. Whenever possible, TT arthrodesis is preferred over TTC arthrodesis to maintain function across the subtalar joint and because the union rate is higher for TT arthrodesis. In cases of inadequate talus bone stock, TTC arthrodesis is necessary. Allograft bone or a metal implant is used to maintain length. Any surgeon performing primary TAR should be prepared to treat failures with salvage arthrodesis.

DISCLOSURE

The author had a patent using the 3D printed sphere technology mentioned in this article.

REFERENCES

1. Kim HJ, Suh DH, Yang JH, et al. Total ankle arthroplasty versus ankle arthrodesis for the treatment of end-stage ankle arthritis: a meta-analysis of comparative studies. Int Orthop 2017;41(1):101–9.
2. Stavrakis AI, SooHoo NF. Trends in complication rates following ankle arthrodesis and total ankle replacement. J Bone Joint Surg Am 2016;98(17):1453–8.
3. Adams SB Jr, Demetracopoulos CA, Queen RM, et al. Early to mid-term results of fixed-bearing total ankle arthroplasty with a modular intramedullary tibial component. J Bone Joint Surg Am 2014;96(23):1983–9.
4. Easley ME, Adams SB Jr, Hembree WC, et al. Results of total ankle arthroplasty. J Bone Joint Surg Am 2011;93(15):1455–68.
5. Harston A, Lazarides AL, Adams SB Jr, et al. Midterm outcomes of a fixed-bearing total ankle arthroplasty with deformity analysis. Foot Ankle Int 2017; 38(12):1295–300.
6. Lewis JS Jr, Green CL, Adams SB Jr, et al. Comparison of first- and second-generation fixed-bearing total ankle arthroplasty using a modular intramedullary tibial component. Foot Ankle Int 2015;36(8):881–90.
7. Schweitzer KM Jr, Adams SB Jr, Easley ME, et al. Total ankle arthroplasty with a modern fixed-bearing system: the salto talaris prosthesis. JBJS Essent Surg Tech 2014;3(3):e18.
8. Schweitzer KM, Adams SB, Viens NA, et al. Early prospective clinical results of a modern fixed-bearing total ankle arthroplasty. J Bone Joint Surg Am 2013;95(11): 1002–11.

9. Stewart MG, Green CL, Adams SB Jr, et al. Midterm results of the salto talaris total ankle arthroplasty. Foot Ankle Int 2017;38(11):1215–21.

10. Labek G, Thaler M, Janda W, et al. Revision rates after total joint replacement: cumulative results from worldwide joint register datasets. J Bone Joint Surg Br 2011; 93(3):293–7.

11. Escudero MI, Le V, Barahona M, et al. Total ankle arthroplasty survival and risk factors for failure. Foot Ankle Int 2019. 1071100719849084.

12. Cody EA, Bejarano-Pineda L, Lachman JR, et al. Risk factors for failure of total ankle arthroplasty with a minimum five years of follow-up. Foot Ankle Int 2019; 40(3):249–58.

13. Ellington JK, Gupta S, Myerson MS. Management of failures of total ankle replacement with the agility total ankle arthroplasty. J Bone Joint Surg Am 2013;95(23):2112–8.

14. Ajis A, Tan KJ, Myerson MS. Ankle arthrodesis vs TTC arthrodesis: patient outcomes, satisfaction, and return to activity. Foot Ankle Int 2013;34(5):657–65.

15. Kruidenier J, van der Plaat LW, Sierevelt IN, et al. Ankle fusion after failed ankle replacement in rheumatic and non-rheumatic patients. Foot Ankle Surg 2019; 25(5):589–93.

16. Jeng CL, Campbell JT, Tang EY, et al. Tibiotalocalcaneal arthrodesis with bulk femoral head allograft for salvage of large defects in the ankle. Foot Ankle Int 2013;34(9):1256–66.

17. Sagherian BH, Claridge RJ. Salvage of failed total ankle replacement using tantalum trabecular metal: case series. Foot Ankle Int 2015;36(3):318–24.

18. Aubret S, Merlini L, Fessy M, et al. Poor outcomes of fusion with Trabecular metal implants after failed total ankle replacement: early results in 11 patients. Orthop Traumatol Surg Res 2018;104(2):231–7.

19. Dekker TJ, Steele JR, Federer AE, et al. Use of patient-specific 3D-printed titanium implants for complex foot and ankle limb salvage, deformity correction, and arthrodesis procedures. Foot Ankle Int 2018;39(8):916–21.

20. Lachman JR, Ramos JA, DeOrio JK, et al. Outcomes of acute hematogenous periprosthetic joint infection in total ankle arthroplasty treated with irrigation, debridement, and polyethylene exchange. Foot Ankle Int 2018;39(11):1266–71.

21. Shi GG, Huh J, Gross CE, et al. Total ankle arthroplasty following prior infection about the ankle. Foot Ankle Int 2015;36(12):1425–9.

22. Glazebrook MA, Arsenault K, Dunbar M. Evidence-based classification of complications in total ankle arthroplasty. Foot Ankle Int 2009;30(10):945–9.

23. Whalen JL, Spelsberg SC, Murray P. Wound breakdown after total ankle arthroplasty. Foot Ankle Int 2010;31(4):301–5.

24. Gross C, Erickson BJ, Adams SB, et al. Ankle arthrodesis after failed total ankle replacement: a systematic review of the literature. Foot Ankle Spec 2015;8(2): 143–51.

25. Rahm S, Klammer G, Benninger E, et al. Inferior results of salvage arthrodesis after failed ankle replacement compared to primary arthrodesis. Foot Ankle Int 2015;36(4):349–59.

26. Kamrad I, Henricson A, Magnusson H, et al. Outcome after salvage arthrodesis for failed total ankle replacement. Foot Ankle Int 2016;37(3):255–61.

27. Deleu PA, Devos Bevernage B, Maldague P, et al. Arthrodesis after failed total ankle replacement. Foot Ankle Int 2014;35(6):549–57.

28. Ali AA, Forrester RA, O'Connor P, et al. Revision of failed total ankle arthroplasty to a hindfoot fusion: 23 consecutive cases using the Phoenix nail. Bone Joint J 2018; 100-B(4):475–9.

29. Halverson AL, Goss DA Jr, Berlet GC. Ankle arthrodesis with structural grafts can work for the salvage of failed total ankle arthroplasty. Foot Ankle Spec 2019. 1938640019843317.
30. McCoy TH, Goldman V, Fragomen AT, et al. Circular external fixator-assisted ankle arthrodesis following failed total ankle arthroplasty. Foot Ankle Int 2012; 33(11):947–55.
31. Doets HC, Zurcher AW. Salvage arthrodesis for failed total ankle arthroplasty. Acta Orthop 2010;81(1):142–7.

Treatment of Ankle and Hindfoot Charcot Arthropathy

Michael S. Pinzur, MD

KEYWORDS

- Charcot foot • Diabetic • Deformity • Ankle • Hindfoot

KEY POINTS

- Charcot foot arthropathy at the level of the hindfoot and ankle poses more complex problems than deformity at the level of the midfoot.
- Favorable clinical outcomes require reestablishment of a normal relationship between the talus and the forefoot and the talus and the calcaneus.
- Deformity at the level of the ankle must be corrected in a stable fashion.

INTRODUCTION

A 3-year observational investigation by the American Orthopedic Foot and Ankle Society Charcot Study Group serves as the foundation for the current interest in surgical correction of the acquired deformity associated with Charcot foot arthropathy.[1] This investigation demonstrated that the historic method of accommodative bracing of the acquired deformity was often successful in resolving infection, but was universally unsuccessful in improving the actual quality of life in affected individuals.[1–3] The current indications for surgical correction of the acquired Charcot foot deformity are clinically and radiographically nonplantigrade deformity with or without an open wound and osteomyelitis. Most experts now also perform surgical correction for plantigrade "rocker-bottom" deformity with instability due to a painful "nonunion" at the location of the disease process.[4–10] The current goals of surgical treatment are (1) resolution of infection, (2) limb salvage, and (3) restoration of a plantigrade "shoeable" foot. The desired clinical outcome is restoration of a foot that is ulcer-free and infection-free, clinically and radiographically plantigrade, and able to allow community ambulation with a commercially available depth-inlay (diabetic) shoe and custom accommodative foot orthosis.[4,10–12]

Several investigators have demonstrated a high rate of successful clinical outcomes when the deformity is located in the midfoot between the talonavicular joint and the

Loyola University Health System, 2160 South First Avenue, Maywood, IL 60153, USA
E-mail address: mpinzu1@lumc.edu

Foot Ankle Clin N Am 25 (2020) 293–303
https://doi.org/10.1016/j.fcl.2020.02.010
1083-7515/20/© 2020 Elsevier Inc. All rights reserved.

foot.theclinics.com

tarsal metatarsal levels. These relatively simple deformity patterns are treated with tendon lengthening of dynamically deforming motor units and wedge-resection osteotomy at the apex of the deformity. Favorable clinical outcomes have been achieved with either intramedullary beaming or circular external fixation.[5,7,8,10,12] The ability to achieve a favorable clinical outcome and avoid complications is greatly decreased when the deformity is proximal to the talonavicular joint and involves the talocalcaneal or tibiotalar (ankle) joints.[8–10] The goal of this review was to provide the reader a clinical algorithm to tackle these more complex deformities.

WHY IS THE ANKLE DIFFERENT?

During normal human walking, initial loading occurs in the center of the heel, progresses up the middle of the foot, and exits under the hallux metatarsophalangeal joint at push-off (**Fig. 1**A, B). Acquired midfoot deformity transfers the weight-bearing load at the transition of mid-stance to push-off to either the medial surface of the foot

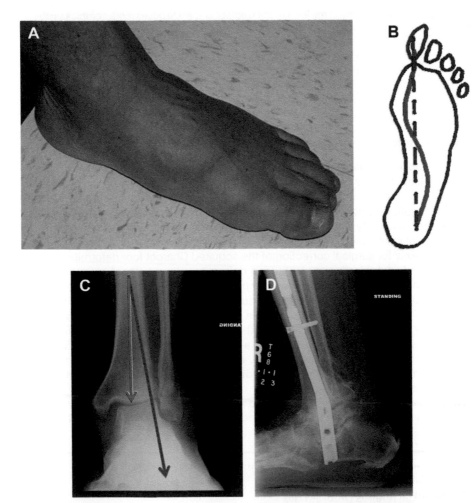

Fig. 1. A 54-year-old woman with body mass index of 47.1. (*A*) Appearance of preoperative foot. (*B*) Simulated weight bearing. Radiographs (*C, D*) at 1 year following surgery.

underlying an exposed head of the talus, or the lateral border of the foot. Either of these deformity patterns creates a bony prominence underneath skin not "designed" for weight bearing at the time of maximal loading. Restoration of a more normal loading pattern is achieved with a wedge-resection osteotomy at the apex of the deformity.[13,14] Normal loading of the ankle joint occurs through the center of the ankle joint. Progressive deformity at the ankle provides a mechanical advantage for a deforming force that accentuates the deformity (**Fig. 1**C).[15,16] A small deformity at the ankle joint level is likely to progress, leading to nonplantigrade loading, instability, and tissue breakdown. This leads to complex late varus and valgus deformities, depending on the direction of loading, that is, pattern, of the original deforming force.

A less common subtalar pattern presents with a varus hindfoot deformity (**Fig. 2**). These patients generally have open wounds with osteomyelitis. As with the valgus pattern, the first step is percutaneous tendon Achilles lengthening. Soft tissue release in this patient group is accomplished by step-cut or fractional lengthening of the

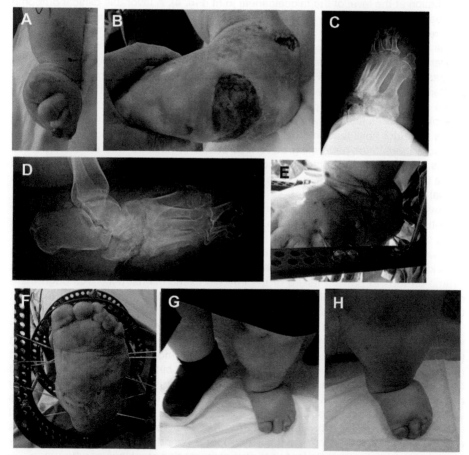

Fig. 2. (*A, B*) This 56-year-old morbidly obese woman presented with the varus deformity with an open wound and osteomyelitis. (*C, D*) Radiographs. She underwent single-stage debridement of the osteomyelitis, correction of the deformity, and maintenance of the correction with a 3-level static circular external fixator. (*E, F*) Photographs at 2 weeks after surgery, and (*G, H*) at 2 years.

posterior tibialis, flexor hallucis longus, and flexor digitorum longus tendons. This is following by debridement of the osteomyelitis and dorsolateral-based wedge-resection osteotomy to create a plantigrade foot. Provisional fixation is accomplished with stout smooth Steinman pins. The correction is then maintained with a 3-level static circular external fixator. Patients receive 6 weeks of culture-specific antibiotic therapy. The frame is removed at 12 weeks (see **Fig. 2**).

DEFORMITY LIMITED TO THE TALOCALCANEAL JOINT

This is a "hybrid" deformity that combines elements of a relatively straightforward midfoot deformity and a more complex ankle-hindfoot deformity. In this hybrid deformity pattern, the ankle joint maintains its structural and radiographic integrity. These patients generally present clinically with a severe valgus deformity (**Fig. 3**).[8] Weight-bearing radiographs of the foot and ankle characteristically demonstrate a normal relationship between the tibia and talus, with severe subluxation or complete lateral dislocation at the level of the talocalcaneal joint (**Fig. 4**). A favorable clinical outcome can be achieved only when a stable relationship between the talus and calcaneus is restored.

The first step is a soft tissue release. This Is accomplished by either a triple hemisection lengthening of the Achilles tendon or a fractional musculotendinous lengthening of the gastrocnemius muscle. Fractional or step-cut lengthening of the peroneal tendons is often necessary to both decrease the dynamic deforming force and facilitate access to the deformity. Using the principle of approaching the deformity at its apex, exposure of the talocalcaneal joint is best achieved with a medial incision along the course of the posterior tibial tendon. This surgical approach has been popularized by Jeng and colleagues[17] for performing triple arthrodesis in patients with severe rigid pes valgus. Bony sacrifice to achieve reduction of the talocalcaneal joint should be skewed to the talus, but care should be taken to maintain a stable ankle joint that will retain a crucial motion segment.

Provisional fixation can be accomplished with stout percutaneous large-bore smooth Steinman pins. Neutralization is then most easily accomplished with a 3-level static circular external fixator (**Fig. 5**). If there is a concern for loss of fixation, the provisional fixation wires can be maintained. Some investigators have now popularized a "hybrid" approach to this deformity pattern, using some form of internal fixation with a "frame on top" to prevent failure of the internal fixation construct.[18] Although there have been case reports of gradual correction in this patient population, I feel that the risks outweigh the benefits, and therefore always favor acute correction.

These patients are often morbidly obese, making it very difficult for them to avoid weight bearing. A "frame shoe" can be fabricated to allow partial weight bearing (**Fig. 6**). A computed tomography scan is performed no earlier than 12 weeks and repeated monthly until there is radiographic evidence of fusion of between one-third and one-half of the fusion surface. The circular frame is removed in the operating room with mild sedation. A cast or fracture boot is then used until swelling subsides and fitting of therapeutic footwear can be accomplished. Although the ultimate goal is therapeutic footwear without an ankle foot orthosis, the author frequently advises a short ankle foot orthosis ("Arizona" - type) for a period of 6 months, when a long-term decision on therapeutic footwear and compression stockings can be made.

A less common subtalar pattern presents with a varus hindfoot deformity (see **Fig. 2**). These patients generally have open wounds with osteomyelitis. As with the valgus pattern, the first step is percutaneous tendon Achilles lengthening. Soft tissue release in this patient group is accomplished by step-cut or fractional lengthening of

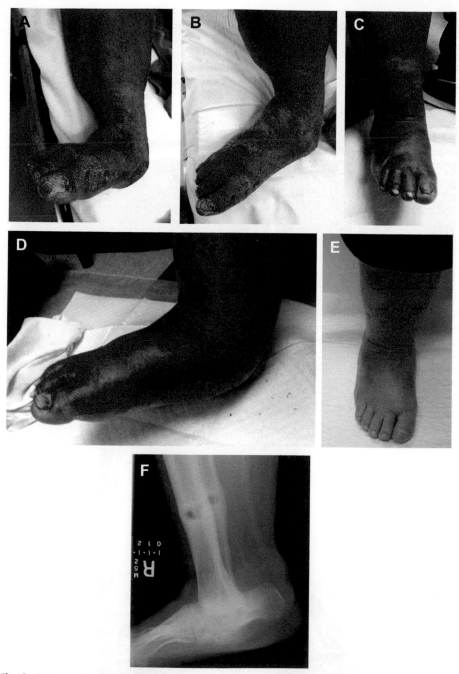

Fig. 3. Preoperative weight-bearing radiographs. (*A*). On this weight-bearing anterior-posterior radiograph, the calcaneus is dislocated laterally from underneath the talus. (*B, C*). The weight-bearing anterior-posterior radiograph of the foot demonstrates lateral dislocation of the talocalcaneal joint. Superimposition of the talus on the calcaneus supports the complete dislocation of the joint. (*D, E, F*). Radiographs at 1 year following surgery.

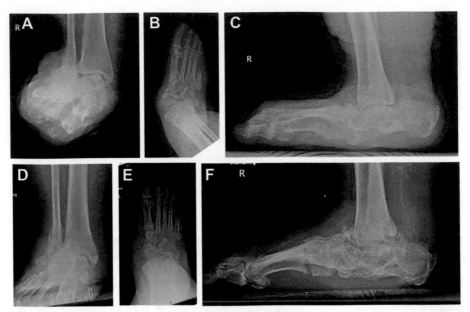

Fig. 4. Preoperative weight-bearing radiographs in a diabetic patient with a midfoot level DISLOCATION pattern Charcot foot arthropathy. (*A*) A weight-bearing anterior-posterior radiograph of the ankle demonstrates complete lateral dislocation of the calcaneus on the talus. (*B*) The anterior-posterior radiograph of the foot demonstrates the severe valgus deformity. (*C*) The magnitude of the deformity is best appreciated on the lateral radiograph where there is overlap of the talus and calcaneus, indicating complete dislocation. (*D, E, F*) Radiographs at 1 year demonstrate greatly improved alignment at the expense of bone from the undersurface of the talus.

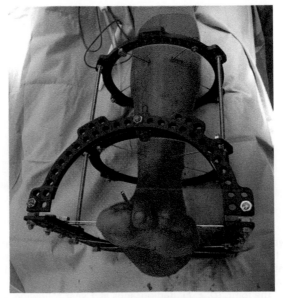

Fig. 5. Provisional fixation was accomplished with stout smooth pins. Neutralization is accomplished with a 3-level static circular external fixator.

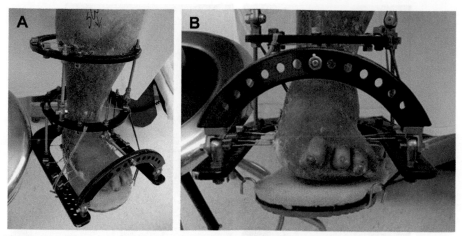

Fig. 6. (*A, B*) A modified "frame" shoe is fashioned from a padded cast shoe to allow the patients to partially weight bear.

the posterior tibialis, flexor hallucis longus, and flexor digitorum longus tendons. This is following by debridement of the osteomyelitis and dorsolateral-based wedge-resection osteotomy to create a plantigrade foot. Provisional fixation is accomplished with stout smooth Steinman pins. The correction is then maintained with a 3-level static circular external fixator. Patients receive 6 weeks of culture-specific antibiotic therapy. The frame is removed at 12 weeks (see **Fig. 2**).[19]

ANKLE JOINT INVOLVEMENT WITHOUT INFECTION

Connolly and Csencsitz,[20] in 1998, reported on a series of neuropathic patients who underwent amputation following ankle fracture. It is now appreciated that because of the applied forces discussed earlier, patients with deformity that involves the ankle joint are less likely to achieve a favorable clinical outcome and avoid complication.[7–9] Stability and weight-bearing alignment that approaches the normal are essential to achieve a favorable clinical outcome. The hormonal-based osteoporosis and poor

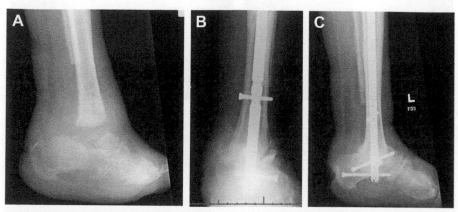

Fig. 7. (*A*) This diabetic patient absorbed much of the talus following the development of a neuropathic ankle. (*B, C*) A tibiotalocalcaneal arthrodesis created a stable well aligned limb for walking.

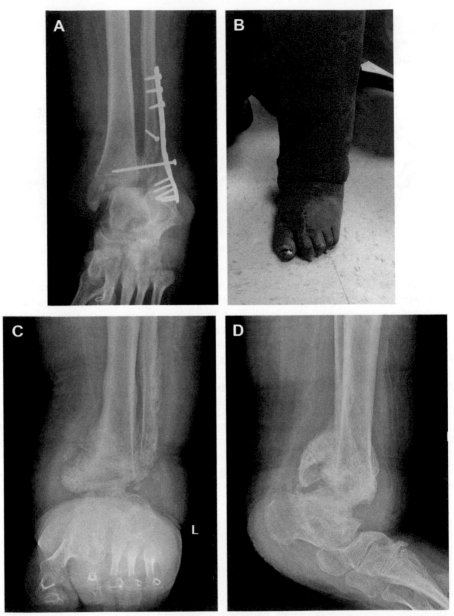

Fig. 8. (*A*) This 49-year-old morbidly obese diabetic woman developed an infected neuro-pathic ankle following an attempt at surgical stabilization of an unstable ankle fracture. In a single-staged procedure, the implants and infected bone were removed, the deformity was corrected with corrective osteotomy, and a standard ankle fusion circular frame was used to maintain the corrected position until bony union. (*B–D*). The patient was stable clin-ically and radiographically at 1 year.

bone quality that limits the ability to achieve a stable bony construct to perform a standard ankle fusion has influenced most experts to favor a retrograde locked intra-medullary nail as the method of choice to achieve stable fixation, in the absence of infection.

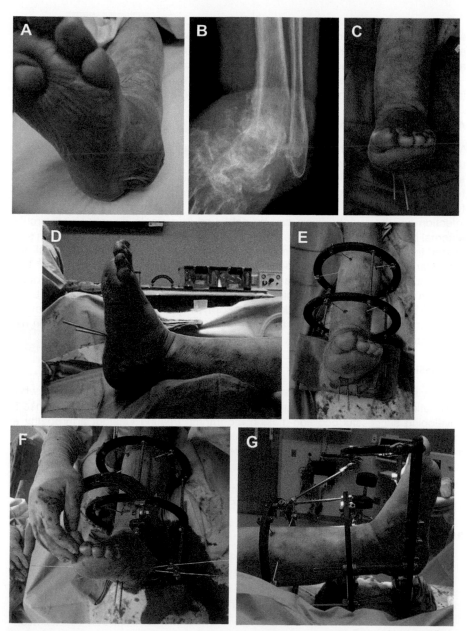

Fig. 9. (*A, B*) This 64-year-old woman developed an infected neuropathic ankle following a low-energy fracture. The medial malleolus was absorbed, leading to a pressure ulcer and seeding of the joint. (*C, D*) Following debridement from a lateral transmalleolar approach, provisional fixation was accomplished with stout smooth wires. (*E*) A tibial mounting block, consisting of 2 connected circular rings was applied to the tibial "reference" segment. (*F*) A closed foot ring was attached to the foot, which acts as the "moving" segment. (*G*) Threaded rods are used to connect, and compress, the "moving" segment to the "reference" segment.

Surgical access to the deformity is most readily achieved by approaching the ankle at the apex of the deformity. A transmalleolar approach is favored when the surgical access is medial or lateral. Arthrodesis of the talocalcaneal joint is optional. Allografts are avoided to decrease the risk for bony collapse or foreign body infection.

Postoperatively, patients are allowed to bear weight in a total contact cast until there is clinical and radiographic evidence of successful arthrodesis (**Fig. 7**).

ANKLE JOINT INVOLVEMENT WITH INFECTION

Most neuropathic (Charcot) ankles develop following fracture. Many are secondary to unsuccessful attempts at open reduction (**Fig. 8**). The steps to achieve successful limb salvage include resolution of infection followed by corrective osteotomy/ankle fusion to create a stable plantigrade limb. Although the historic treatment has advocated performing this treatment in stages, it has now been demonstrated that resolution of infection and bony arthrodesis can be achieved in a single surgery when circular external fixation is used to achieve a stable contruct.[19] More recently, it has been suggested that a hybrid construct combining an antibiotic-coated intramedullary nail and a circular external fixator has the potential to achieve single-stage limb salvage.[18] That said, a successful limb salvage can be accomplished by single-stage resection of the infection and ankle fusion with a circular external fixator with or without hybrid internal fixtion.[9] The use of locally introduced vancomycin powder in the wound following debridement and before fixation appears to have the potential to decrease the risk for infection (**Fig. 9**).

DISCUSSION

As early as 1998, Connolly and Csencsitz[20] realized the high risk for amputation when a diabetic patient develops a neuropathic ankle. Based on the experience gained in developing successful decision-making algorithms treating Charcot arthropathy at the level of the midfoot, we are now developing successful strategies for salvaging a stable limb when the neuropathic process attacks the hindfoot or ankle.

DISCLOSURE

The author is a consultant on this topic to Stryker USA.

REFERENCES

1. Dhawan V, Spratt KF, Pinzur MS, et al. Reliability of AOFAS diabetic foot questionnaire in Charcot arthropathy: stability, internal consistency and measurable difference. Foot Ankle Int 2005;26(9):717–31.
2. Raspovic KR, Wukich DK. Self-reported quality of life in patients with diabetes: a comparison of patients with and without Charcot neuroarthropathy. Foot Ankle Int 2014;35(10):195–200.
3. Kroin E, Schiff AP, Pinzur MS, et al. Functional impairment of patients undergoing surgical correction for Charcot foot arthropathy. Foot Ankle Int 2017;38(7):705–9.
4. Rogers LC, Frykberg RG, Armstrong DG, et al. The diabetic Charcot foot syndrome: a report of the joint task force on the Charcot foot by the American Diabetes Association and the American Podiatric Medical Association. Diabetes Care 2011;34:2123–9.
5. Sammarco VJ, Sammarco GJ, Walker EW, et al. Midtarsal arthrodesis in treatment of Charcot midfoot arthropathy. J Bone Joint Surg Am 2009;91(1):80–91.

6. Ford SE, Cohen BE, Davis WH, et al. Clinical outcomes and complications of mid-foot Charcot reconstruction with intramedullary beaming. Foot Ankle Int 2019; 40(1):18–23.
7. Pinzur MS. Neutral ring fixation for high risk non-plantigrade Charcot midfoot deformity. Foot Ankle Int 2007;28(9):961–6.
8. Pinzur MS, Schiff AP. Deformity and clinical outcomes following surgical correction of Charcot foot: a new classification with implications for treatment. Foot Ankle Int 2018;39(3):265–70.
9. Harkins E, Murphy M, Schneider A, et al. Deformity and clinical outcomes following surgical correction of Charcot ankle. Foot Ankle Int 2019;40(2):145–51.
10. Jones C, McCormick J, Pinzur MS. Surgical treatment of Charcot foot. In: Instructional course lectures of the American Academy of Orthopaedic Surgeons, 67 2018;. p. 255–67.
11. Strotman P, Reif TJ, Pinzur MS. Current concepts: Charcot arthropathy of the foot and ankle. Foot Ankle Int 2016;37(11):1255–63.
12. Kroin E, Chaharbakhshi EO, Schiff A, et al. Improvement in quality of life following surgical correction of midtarsal Charcot foot deformity. Foot Ankle Int 2018;39(7): 808–11.
13. Bevan WP, Tomlinson MP. Radiographic measure as a predictor of ulcer formation in diabetic Charcot midfoot. Foot Ankle Int 2008;29:568–73.
14. Pinzur MS. Surgical vs. accommodative treatment for Charcot arthropathy of the midfoot. Foot Ankle Int 2004;25:545–9.
15. Hastings MK, Johnson JE, Strube MJ, et al. Progression of foot deformity in Charcot neuropathic osteoarthropathy. J Bone Joint Surg Am 2013;95A:1206–13.
16. Wukich DK, Raspovic KM, Hobizal KB, et al. Radiographic analysis of diabetic midfoot Charcot neuroarthropathy with and without midfoot ulceration. Foot Ankle Int 2014;35(11):1108–15.
17. Jeng CL, Vora AM, Myerson MS. The medial approach to triple arthrodesis. Indications and technique for management of rigid valgus deformities in high-risk patients. Foot Ankle Clin 2005;10(3):515–21.
18. Tomczak C, Beaman D, Perkins S. Combined intramedullary nail coated with antibiotic-containing cement and ring fixation for limb salvage in the severely deformed, infected neuroarthropathic ankle. Foot Ankle Int 2019;40(1):48–55.
19. Pinzur MS, Gil J, Belmares J. Treatment of osteomyelitis in Charcot foot with single stage resection of infection, correction of deformity and maintenance with ring fixation. Foot Ankle Int 2012;33(12):1069–74.
20. Connolly JF, Csencsitz TA. Limb threatening neuropathic complications from ankle fractures in patients with diabetes. Clin Orthop 1998;348:212–9.

Managing the Complex Cavus Foot Deformity

Mark S. Myerson, MD[a], C. Lucas Myerson, MD[b],*

KEYWORDS

- Cavus foot • Deformity • Correction

KEY POINTS

- In carefully selected cases, the rigid cavovarus foot may be corrected with a combination of osteotomies and tendon transfers rather than a triple arthrodesis.
- In a foot with multiplanar deformity, multiple levels of arthrodesis and osteotomies need to be considered to correct the deformity in all planes.
- A deformity secondary to progressive peripheral neuropathy cannot reliably be corrected and maintained with a triple arthrodesis alone.
- It is essential to address the hindfoot before addressing deformity in the midfoot or forefoot.
- Soft tissue balancing must be performed to prevent recurrence and achieve a plantigrade foot.

INTRODUCTION

This article describes approaches to and the management of complex cavus foot deformities. Correction of rigid multiplanar deformities can be very challenging, given the presence of skeletal deformities in multiple planes and combined with a varying degree of muscle imbalance. The complexity of these cases always requires a case-by-case approach. Some of the cases presented here occur in patients who have previously undergone surgical management for their deformity, several of which are complicated by additional deformities. With a firm understanding and application of the principles of deformity correction, however, one may reliably offer satisfactory results.

The principles of deformity correction are varied, but can be summarized into a few salient points.

- Osteotomies (or arthrodesis) must be performed at the apex of deformity.
- Tendon transfers must be performed to improve muscle imbalance.

[a] Steps2Walk, Baltimore, MD 21230, USA; [b] Department of Orthopaedic Surgery, Penn Medicine, 3737 Market Street, Philadelphia, PA 19104, USA
* Corresponding author.
E-mail address: lucasmyerson@gmail.com

Foot Ankle Clin N Am 25 (2020) 305–317
https://doi.org/10.1016/j.fcl.2020.02.006
1083-7515/20/© 2020 Elsevier Inc. All rights reserved.

- A plantar fascia release is invariably performed.
- A biplanar or triplanar calcaneal osteotomy may be added to a hindfoot arthrodesis.
- Peroneus longus-to-brevis transfer is useful, particularly in the younger patient.
- A posterior tibial tendon transfer or tenotomy is generally required.
- Resection of the base of the fifth metatarsal is necessary for fixed midfoot varus.
- Occasionally osteotomy of the first metatarsal is required.

All of the cases in this article presented with a rigid deformity, which traditionally has relied on triple arthrodesis for correction. However, we have found that, in selected cases, even though the foot is very rigid, correction and the achievement of a planti-grade foot through a variety of osteotomies in combination with tendon transfers can be performed. A triple arthrodesis is not always necessary even in the presence of a rigid deformity. With each of these cases, we start by identifying the key points that should be brought up in the presurgical evaluation. Then, we move on to a discussion of surgical options for each deformity.

CAVOEQUINUS DEFORMITY

The first case we present is that of a patient with a unilateral cavoequinus deformity (**Fig. 1**A, B). In a patient with a unilateral deformity, the deformity may be the result of poliomyelitis, congenital spinal cord lesions, spinocerebellar degeneration, or a va-riety of post-traumatic disorders. In this particular case, this young man sustained an injury to the limb producing a traumatic nerve injury. Other causes of a unilateral post-traumatic deformity may be the result of scarring in the deep posterior compartment of the leg after a compartment syndrome or sciatic or peroneal nerve injury. Identifying the etiology is important to understand how, and to what extent, surgical intervention will mitigate the progression of the deformity.

The cavoequinus deformity in this case is fairly typical of a nerve injury. We can observe significant deformity of the hindfoot, with an elevated calcaneal pitch angle and significant varus (see **Fig. 1**A, B). In addition to these deformities of the hindfoot, there is deformity in the midfoot. The entire midfoot has derotated and the fifth meta-tarsal can be seen lying underneath the cuboid (**Fig. 1**C–E). Finally, there is significant claw toe deformity of the forefoot, which is not addressed in this article.

The triple arthrodesis is a safe and reliable option for management of this severe, rigid cavus deformity. We do not agree with the findings of Wetmore and Drennan,[1] who evaluated 16 patients who had Charcot-Marie-Tooth disease and underwent a tri-ple arthrodesis, most of them bilaterally. The average age at the time of operation was 15 years, and the average length of follow-up was 21 years. Of the 30 feet, the result in 2 was rated excellent, in 5 good, in 9 fair, and in 14 poor. Six limbs had an arthrodesis of the ankle for degenerative joint disease. Progressive muscle imbalance resulted in recurrent cavovarus deformity in 7 feet that initially had had satisfactory alignment. Degenerative changes of the ankle and joints of the midpart of the foot were noted radiographically in 23 feet. We believe that the large number of unsatisfactory long-term results in these patients who had undergone a triple arthrodesis for deformity was the result of inadequate muscle balance at the time of the triple arthrodesis. One cannot rely on a triple arthrodesis to correct and maintain the correction of a deformity in the setting of a deformity that is secondary to progressive peripheral neu-ropathy. Clearly, this group of patients with a neuromuscular etiology differs from those in patients who have poliomyelitis, who retain normal sensation and have a per-manent but stable muscle imbalance. If performed in isolation, a triple arthrodesis re-sults in predictable failure because the arthrodesis must be accompanied by

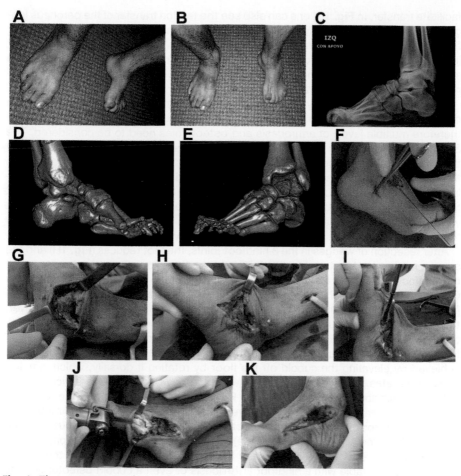

Fig. 1. The appearance of a severe unilateral rigid deformity caused by peripheral nerve injury (*A, B*). Radiograph and 3-dimensional computed tomography reconstruction confirm the magnitude of the deformity in particular the position of the fifth metatarsal under the cuboid (*C–E*). A plantar fasciotomy is performed (*F*), followed by lateral exposure of all 3 joints (*G*). The triple arthrodesis is performed through a single lateral incision with realignment and fixation commencing laterally (*H, I*). Owing to persistent pressure under the fifth metatarsal base, it was resected with a saw, noting a soft skin pad after the ostectomy (*J, K*).

additional procedures to address the muscle imbalance and soft tissue contractures. These factors include a combination of plantar fasciotomy, tenotomy or transfer of the posterior tibial tendon, as well as a transfer of the peroneus longus to brevis.

The release of the plantar fascia is usually the first procedure we perform, because correction of the calcaneus can otherwise be challenging owing to soft tissue contracture. In **Fig. 1**F, one can see that the plantar fascia is released through a 1 cm medial longitudinal incision adjacent to the heel. In this case, the posterior tibial tendon (PTT) has already been dissected for transfer. The incision used for transfer of the PTT should be planned carefully in a patient such as this, who is expected to require additional incisions for the various bony procedures. One can see in **Fig. 1**F that the PTT has been exposed and a 2-0 suture has been inserted into the end of the tendon to facilitate transfer. In **Fig. 1**G, one can also see the tendon transfer of the peroneus longus to brevis, which not only improves eversion strength, but decrease the plantar flexion–deforming force on the first metatarsal as well. The technique for this transfer involves suturing both tendons together before cutting the longus to achieve the appropriate tension. If the longus is cut before suture, it is more difficult to find the correct resting tension for the transfer.

A key principle of deformity correction is performing the correction at the apex of the deformity(ies). In a foot with multiplanar deformity, multiple apices are present and therefore multiple levels of arthrodesis and osteotomies need to be considered. The 3-dimensional computed tomography reconstructions (see **Fig. 1**D, E) show deformity through the calcaneocuboid (CC), subtalar and talonavicular joints. Wedge resections through all 3 joints beginning at the CC joint (see **Fig. 1**G) permits reduction of the subluxated CC joint and derotation of the midfoot. In the same **Fig. 1**G, one can see that the PTT has been transferred from the medial to the lateral compartment through a window created in the interosseous membrane. Ideally, it should be the muscle belly that crosses the window rather than the tendon to avoid adhesions.

After resection of wedges in the 3 hindfoot joints, the foot reduces (**Fig. 1**H) and the screws are inserted first across the CC and then the talonavicular joints. We find it more effective to insert the first screw at the apex of the deformity, in this case the CC joint (**Fig. 1**I). Note that there is considerable pressure from the thumb under the fifth metatarsal attempting to elevate it; the CC joint is fixed in position. However, the prominent callosity underneath the base of the fifth metatarsal persisted caused, as noted elsewhere in this article, by pressure overload on the lateral border of the foot, which failed to derotate with the triple arthrodesis. The rotatory maneuver is achieved by elevating the cuboid off the floor by rotating it dorsally, which simultaneously elevates the fifth metatarsal. One should have been able to anticipate this in the 3-dimensional reconstruction (see **Fig. 1**D, E) because the fifth metatarsal is completely under the cuboid. This state frequently causes overload of the metatarsal and can be associated with a stress fracture of the metatarsal shaft (usually at the junction of the metaphysis and diaphysis), which can be painful for the patient and needs to be corrected. The derotation of the fifth metatarsal underneath the cuboid will not be correctable with a hindfoot arthrodesis or even a cuboid osteotomy if the metatarsal is completely fixed in this position under the cuboid. To sufficiently correct this deformity, one must directly address the fifth metatarsal with a partial resection of the base.[2] The resection should be performed through an extension of the incision on the lateral aspect of the foot used for the previous osteotomies. The incision should run from the base of the fifth metatarsal distally along the dorsal aspect of the metatarsal shaft. An oblique saw cut is made from distal to proximal and lateral to medial to reduce the bony protrusion caused by the base of the fifth metatarsal (**Fig. 1**J). Although the peroneus brevis is useless in this patient, if there is a need to use the brevis tendon, for example, for a nonanatomic ankle ligament reconstruction, the brevis tendon should be anchored near its insertion into the fifth metatarsal, either into soft tissue or into the cuboid. **Fig. 1**K demonstrates that the pressure underneath the base of the fifth metatarsal is no longer present.

CAVUS DEFORMITY ASSOCIATED WITH PRIOR PANTALAR ARTHRODESIS

This case features a cavus joint contracture that has previously undergone treatment with a pantalar arthrodesis for arthrogryposis deformity as an adolescent. The arthrodesis can in theory provide satisfactory results for a hindfoot and ankle deformity, provided that the foot is balanced with the appropriate tendon transfers and accompanied by osteotomies of the midfoot and forefoot. Unfortunately, those procedures were not performed, and the arthrodesis did not sufficiently address the muscle imbalance or the problems of the midfoot and forefoot. The result is a fixed calcaneus of the hindfoot deformity accompanied by rigid supination deformity of the forefoot (**Fig. 2**A, B). The patient presented with pain under the heel, thickened skin of the heel pad, and pain along the lateral border of the foot with no passive dorsiflexion of the hallux.

Invariably, any correction that is done in the hindfoot influences the position of the forefoot, so one must first direct attention to the hindfoot deformity (the calcaneus deformity and the fixed supination deformity with the apex at the talonavicular joint). Before any osteotomy, a complete plantar fasciotomy of both the medial and lateral fascial bands must be performed. In patients who require mobilization of the calcaneal tuberosity, or those who have severe deformity in which the cavus is accompanied by an adductovarus deformity, the insertions of the short flexor muscles must also be entirely removed from the calcaneus. This stripping procedure, first described by Steindler[3] in 1920, involves removal of all plantar soft tissue attachments from the os calcis.

Once the calcaneal tuberosity has been freed of all its attachments, an osteotomy should be performed to address the pitch angle and varus deformity. A triplanar osteotomy that addresses these deformities simultaneously should be used. A closing valgus wedge osteotomy is created to bring the heel out of varus. Then, the tuberosity is shifted laterally and cephalad to improve the weight-bearing axis of the hindfoot and the calcaneal pitch, respectively (**Fig. 2**C, D). Although in this case a triplanar osteotomy is performed, a biplanar osteotomy is often times sufficient when the pitch angle does not require correction.

To address the equinus as well as the supination deformity of the forefoot, a variety of osteotomies of the midfoot must be used (**Fig. 2**F). The plane of correction is dictated not only by the extent of the deformity, but the type of deformity as well. The osteotomy must always be performed at the apex of the deformity, as performed here. Before performing saw cuts, a K wire is introduced to direct the orientation of the saw cut through the talonavicular arthrodesis across to the CC joint (**Fig. 2**G). The saw cut should allow for rotation, that is, protonation as well as dorsiflexion to bring the forefoot out of supination and equinus (**Fig. 2**H). One can visualize this rotation by marking the medial bone with electrocautery in a line perpendicular to the osteotomy. Once the derotation has been completed, the cautery lines should no longer match up easily, confirming the protonation of the osteotomy through the arthrodesis (**Fig. 2**I, J). To correct the cavoequinus midfoot, a wedge must also be removed from the osteotomy to dorsiflex the foot. The osteotomy can be further contoured until sufficient bone has been removed.

The last step of the correction addresses the deformity of the hallux. Noting that there was no passive dorsiflexion of the hallux at the metatarsophalangeal joint (**Fig. 2**K), one has to address the elevatus of the first metatarsal as well as the contracture of the short flexors. An elevated first metatarsal is very unusual in the setting of the cavus foot, particularly when the hindfoot is pronated, which would normally worsen the plantarflexion of the first metatarsal. In this case, however, the anterior tibial tendon was functioning causing the elevatus, and this was transferred laterally into the middle cuneiform (note the small lateral incision in the distal leg in **Fig. 2**C). In this particular patient, the chronic supination deformity of the midfoot causes an impingement or a functional hallux rigidus, which prevents successful dorsiflexion of the first metatarsophalangeal joint. To correct this deformity, a plantar-based wedge must be removed from the tarsometatarsal joint to shorten the hallux and plantarflex

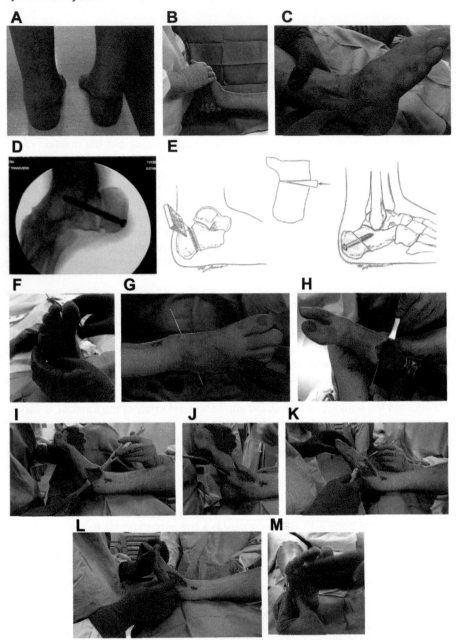

Fig. 2. Management of this cavus foot deformity after pantalar arthrodesis associated with arthrogryposis in a young adult. Note the heel varus and calcaneus and fixed forefoot supination (*A*, *B*), corrected with a biplanar calcaneus osteotomy to shift the heel laterally and cephalad (*C–E*). After the osteotomy, note the fixed forefoot supination with the apex at the talonavicular joint (*F*). The axis of the osteotomy is marked with a guide pin and checked fluorscopically (*G*), and the saw cut initiated medially through the talonavicular fusion (*H*). The foot is pronated (*I*), and fixed with cannulated screws (*J*). The first metatarsal elevatus is blocking passive dorsiflexion of the hallux and a plantar closing wedge arthrodesis is made through the first tarsometatarsal joint (*K*, *L*) successfully achieving a plantigrade forefoot (*M*). (*From* [*E*] Wapner KL. Pes cavus. In: Myerson MS, ed. Foot and Ankle Disorders Volume Two. Philadelphia, PA: W.B. Saunders Company; 2000:919-941; with permission.)

the first metatarsal. This correction can be made through an incision extended dorso-medially spanning the first tarsometatarsal joint (**Fig. 2L**). By a plantarflexion arthrod-esis of the first tarsometatarsal joint, the first metatarsal is positioned in slight equinus, and there is a decrease in the plantar contracture. This maneuver allows the first ray to dorsiflex through the metatarsophalangeal joint, creating a plantigrade forefoot (**Fig. 2M**).

REVISION OF FAILED CAVUS FOOT DEFORMITY

This case features severe recurrent deformity in a patient with Charcot-Marie-Tooth disease who had previously undergone attempted correction with a triple arthrodesis. One can appreciate the persistent cavovarus deformity in **Fig. 3**A, B, complicated by a stress fracture of the fifth metatarsal, ankle arthritis, and adduction deformity of the midfoot. The high pitch angle of the calcaneus is noted, the persistent varus of the hindfoot, and the rotation of the midfoot, in particular with the fifth metatarsal close to the floor. The metatarsals are all stacked one upon the other and the ratio of the height of the medial cuneiform to the floor and the fifth metatarsal to the floor is abnormal.

The original correction may have in part failed owing to the deforming force of the PTT on the midfoot. On examination of this patient, the strength of the posterior tibial muscle was 5 out of 5, the peroneus longus 5 out of 5, the peroneus brevis 2 out of 5, and the anterior tibial muscle 4– out of 5. Correction of this recurrent deformity de-pends on adequate soft tissue balancing, which will includes a plantar fascia release, a PTT transfer through the interosseous membrane to the lateral cuneiform, and a

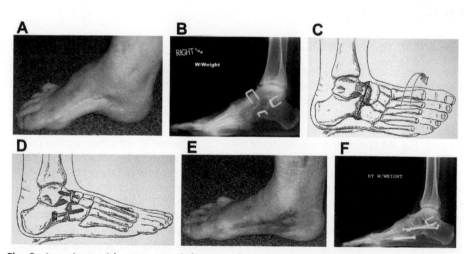

Fig. 3. A patient with recurrent deformity after triple arthrodesis (A, B), corrected with plantar fascia release, posterior tibial tendon transfer, peroneus longus to brevis transfer, revision transverse tarsal arthrodesis, ankle ligament reconstruction, ankle cheilectomy, first metatarsal osteotomy and ORIF fifth metatarsal. The illustration of the wedges and the rota-tion of the transverse tarsal joint (C, D). The final clinical and radiographic appearance (E, F). (From [A, B] Myerson MS, Kadakia AR. Cavus Foot Correction. In: Myerson MS, Kadakia AR. Reconstructive Foot and Ankle Surgery. 3rd ed. Philadelphia, PA: Elsevier; 2019:141-160; with permission; and [C, D] Haddad SL, Myerson MS, Pell RF 4th, et al. Clinical and radiographic outcome of revision surgery for failed triple arthrodesis. Foot Ankle Int. 1997;18(8):489-499; with permission.)

peroneus longus to brevis transfer to reduce the deforming force responsible for the adduction deformity on the midfoot.

Note in **Fig. 3**B that the length of the talus and navicular is very short, which implies that excessive bone was removed from the talonavicular joint when the original arthrodesis was performed. This factor led to shortening of the medial column, which compounded the varus overload of the midfoot. Correction of this overload involves revisiting the midfoot and performing osteotomies through both the CC and talonavicular joints. The transverse tarsal joint cannot be rotated without performing cuts through both of these joints. Laterally, a biplanar wedge is removed to derotate and close down the lateral side of the hindfoot. The apex of the wedge laterally is dorsal and lateral so that the lateral side of the foot can be elevated and rotated while simultaneously correcting the adduction deformity. This principle was originally described by Haddad, Myerson, and colleagues,[4] noting that the correction is always performed at the apex of the deformity, which in this case is distal to the calcaneus and no calcaneus osteotomy was therefore required.

As a result of the persistent hindfoot deformity associated with muscle imbalance, severe varus ankle instability and arthritis developed. These were corrected with an anterior ankle joint cheilectomy and a non anatomic ankle ligament reconstruction. The additional procedures performed to obtain a plantigrade foot were:

- Revision of the triple arthrodesis using a transverse tarsal osteotomy
- Transfer of the PTT
- Transfer of the peroneus longus to the brevis
- Dorsal wedge osteotomy of the first metatarsal

The final clinical and radiographic appearance of the corrected foot is noted in **Fig. 3**E, F.

MANAGING THE SOFT TISSUE CONTRACTURE

This case demonstrates a few of the steps that are involved in a revision of a failed treatment for cavus foot deformity by examining only the soft tissue components of the correction medially for this very severe recurrent cavus foot. As a generalization, the PTT is released, cut, or transferred depending on its strength and mobility. In a case where the PTT is mobile, and modest power (>3+ is present), a transfer is performed. **Fig. 4**A shows the harvesting of the PTT. As noted in our other articles on the cavus foot, failure to transfer the PTT is a common cause for recurrent deformity.[5–7] The tendon is not cut at the navicular tuberosity, but must be detached more distally, including a strip of periosteum over the cuneiform to give a longer length of the tendon for transfer. **Fig. 4**B demonstrates the suture in the PTT and the exposure of the abductor fascia. It is rare that a release of the abductor is necessary, unless the deformity is severe, as noted here, where the adductus deformity was the result of contraction of the abductor fascia compounded by the force of the PTT and the short flexor muscles. It is not appropriate to simply cut the muscle or fascia, and **Fig. 4**C demonstrates the dissection of the abductor fascia, which is then completely cut as far distally as possible removing a segment of the fascia and in this case also cutting the abductor muscle. A plantar fascia release is an integral and essential part of correction of the cavus foot. In the past, we have tried to perform this release with an incision under the arch of the foot where the fascia is easily palpable. However, we recognized that strategy this led to the development of thick scarring on the skin and at times recurrent contracture of the fascia, and we prefer to perform the release as demonstrated in **Fig. 1**F. In this particular case, however, because the entire medial

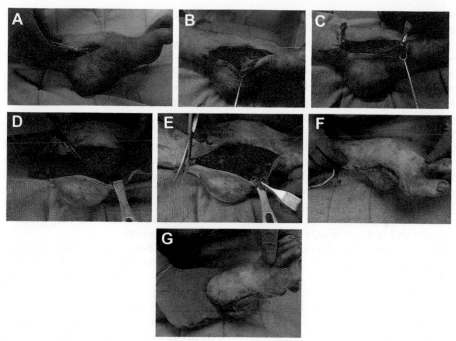

Fig. 4. The sequence of medial soft tissue releases is illustrated with exposure of the posterior tibial tendon (*A*), exposure and removal of the abductor fascia (*B, C*), open plantar fasciectomy (*D, E*), and the final appearance of the foot following the releases in the cavus (*F*) and corrected position (*G*).

aspect of the foot was already exposed, an open approach to resection of the fascia was performed and **Fig.** 4D demonstrates the plantar fasciectomy. In this particular case, excision of a 2-cm strip of plantar fascia was performed through the same incision, which was used to cut the abductor (**Fig.** 4E). For the majority of cavus foot correction procedures, we perform the fasciotomy through separate short incisions at the junction of the normal skin and heel pad more proximally (**Fig.** 1F). The appearance of the foot after the release demonstrates adequate releases and now permits one to proceed with skeletal correction and muscle balancing (**Fig.** 4F, G).

THE USE OF OSTEOTOMY FOR A RIGID DEFORMITY

As noted elsewhere in this article, the impulse to correct a rigid deformity would be with a triple arthrodesis of one variety or another. However, this procedure is not always necessary, and depends on the ability to perform adequate soft tissue releases and balancing, and then to correct the heel varus with osteotomy, followed by a midfoot osteotomy either as described by Cole,[8] or a modified Japas[9] type procedure depending on the apex of the deformity. The calcaneus osteotomy is not performed as a Dwyer type osteotomy,[10] but as that described by Myerson.[11] This procedure is a triplane osteotomy and corrects the varus with a wedge, then moves the tuberosity laterally, and moves the tuberosity cephalad. One has to be careful with the extent of the lateral shift of the calcaneus, because this procedure can cause a tarsal tunnel syndrome.[12] If the varus is severe, we think that a prophylactic release of the tarsal tunnel is useful and can be performed by extending the medial incision for the exposure of the PTT. At times, one can perform the osteotomy and then palpate the skin to determine if it remains soft, and if so a release may not be necessary. This case presented in a 17-year-old with a rigid deformity, the sagittal apex of the deformity was in the naviculocuneiform joints (**Fig. 5**A, B), and a midfoot osteotomy was performed at this level after the calcaneus osteotomy. The latter was a large osteotomy of a 5-mm wedge, but a large lateral shift of 13 mm (**Fig. 5**C). The plantar fascia release and PTT as well as longus to brevis transfer had already been set up, and this was followed by the midfoot osteotomy (**Fig. 5**D, E). A dorsally based wedge is removed from the midfoot. This wedge is maximum over the medial naviculocuneiform joint, and then narrows laterally, until it is a flat cut through the cuboid. Although the wedge tapers from medial to lateral, the wedge is dorsally based, and not medially based. This factor is critical, because a medially based wedge would inappropriately adduct the foot. Once the wedge is removed, the foot is derotated laterally so that the fifth metatarsal and cuboid move as 1 column as they elevate off the floor. The midfoot osteotomies are always fixed with 3-mm pins, which hold the reduction very well and are removed at 4 to 6 weeks in children and 8 weeks in adults.

The same principle is demonstrated in **Figs. 6** and **7**. In **Fig. 6**, this young adult who had a profoundly rigid deformity (see **Fig. 6**A) treated much as described elsewhere in this article (see **Fig. 5**). The PTT was moved, and the peroneal transfer performed, followed by the calcaneus osteotomy (see **Fig. 6**B, C). As in **Fig. 5**, this was a large wedge and lateral shift of 12 mm and one can now note the correction of the heel varus (see **Fig. 6**D), where it is now in valgus. A guide-pin is then inserted across the foot at the apex of the deformity. This insertion may be at the level of the naviculocuneiform joints or through the cuneiforms and cuboid, in this case going directly across the

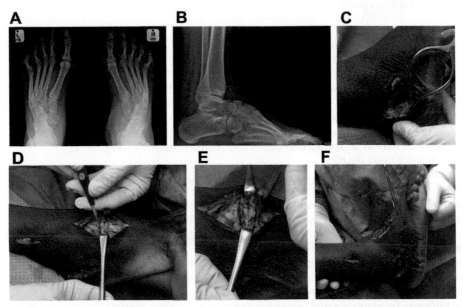

Fig. 5. The correction without triple arthrodesis is demonstrated here in this young patient with a very rigid deformity (*A, B*). After medial release, the triplanar calcaneus osteotomy is performed with a large lateral shift (*C*). This process is followed by a midfoot wedge arthrodesis–osteotomy through the naviculocuneiform joints and cuboid (*D, E*), and the final appearance with pin fixation noted (*F*).

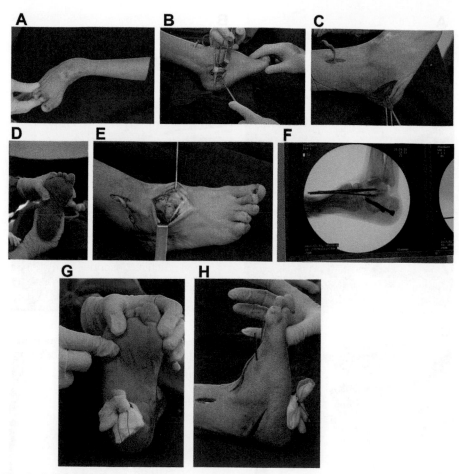

Fig. 6. Correction of a rigid deformity without hindfoot arthrodesis is demonstrated (*A*), first with the medial soft tissue procedures, then peroneus longus to brevis (*B*), an aggressive calcaneus triplane osteotomy (*C*), which positions the hindfoot in valgus but exacerbates the midfoot and forefoot deformity (*D*). The midfoot osteotomy is marked at the apex which here is in the naviculocuneiform joints (*E*, *F*), noting a very well-corrected foot at completion (*G*, *H*).

navicular cuneiform joint and then into the cuboid. In addition to closing the dorsal wedge, the cuneiforms can be translated slightly dorsally to further correct the forefoot equinus (see **Fig. 6**E). The passage of the PTT through the midfoot is demonstrated with a new technique in **Fig. 6**F and G where instead of using an interference screw or a bone anchor, this is a rubber button that is used over a gauze pad. We take the syringe top from a 20 or 30 syringe and then take off the rubber cap and perforate it with 2 clamps to make a hole and then pass sutures attached to the PTT transfer through the rubber cap, which are then tied over a gauze pad on the under surface of the foot. This technique is invaluable and inexpensive in the economically deprived areas where our foundation does the majority of its work. The dorsal shift of the cuneiforms on the navicular is well-demonstrated in **Fig. 7**, a severe rigid deformity (see **Fig. 7**A, B), treated similarly as in **Fig. 6** with a midfoot osteotomy, which highlights the dorsal shift of the cuneiforms to further establish a plantigrade foot (see **Fig. 7**C, D).

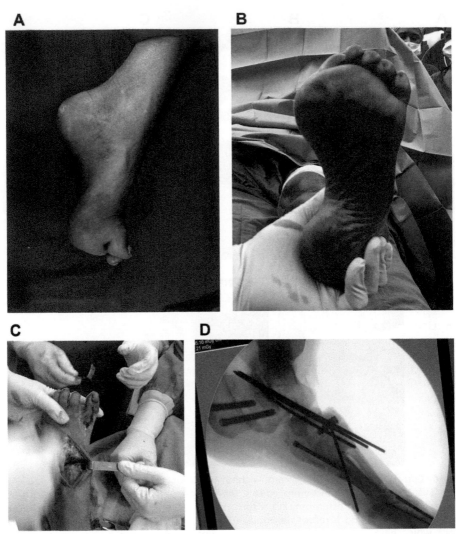

Fig. 7. A profound rigid deformity can be corrected with hindfoot osteotomy and midfoot arthrodesis–osteotomy combined with tendon transfers (*A, B*). Note that after the midfoot procedure, the forefoot is translated dorsally on the navicular and the cuboid is rotated dorsally to produce a plantigrade foot (*C, D*).

SUMMARY

Although the management of severe cavus foot deformity can be treated in a traditional manner with triple arthrodesis or its modifications, one can correct severe deformities with osteotomies instead. It is essential that the calcaneus, midfoot, and then forefoot are addressed. Clearly, a theme that we have emphasized is that, regardless of the magnitude of the deformity, adequate soft tissue balancing must be performed to create a plantigrade foot as well as prevent recurrent deformity. If a triple arthrodesis is selected as the procedure for correction, one may have to add further procedures including resection of the base of the fifth metatarsal, tarsometatarsal arthrodesis or first metatarsal osteotomy, ankle ligament reconstruction and of course tendon transfers.

DISCLOSURE

The authors have nothing to disclose.

REFERENCES

1. Wetmore RS, Drennan JC. Long-term results of triple arthrodesis in Charcot-Marie-Tooth disease. J Bone Joint Surg Am 1989;71:417–22.
2. Shariff R, Myerson MS, Palmanovich E. Resection of the fifth metatarsal base in the severe rigid cavovarus foot. Foot Ankle Int 2014;35:558–65.
3. Steindler A. Stripping of the os calcis. J Bone Joint Surg 1920;2:8–12.
4. Haddad SL, Myerson MS, Pell RF IV, et al. Clinical and radiographic outcome of revision surgery for failed triple arthrodesis. Foot Ankle Int 1997;18:489–99.
5. Myerson MS, Myerson CL. Cavus foot: deciding between osteotomy and arthrodesis. Foot Ankle Clin 2019;24:347–60.
6. Wapner K. The cavus foot. In: Myerson MS, editor. Foot and ankle disorders, vol. 2. Philadelphia: WB Saunders; 2000. p. 919–41.
7. Zide J, Myerson MS. Arthrodesis in managing the cavus foot. Where when and how? Foot Ankle Clin 2013;18:755–67.
8. Cole WH. The treatment of claw-foot. JBJS 1940;22:895–908.
9. Japas LM. Surgical treatment of pes cavus by tarsal V-osteotomy: preliminary report. J Bone Joint Surg Am 1968;50:927–44.
10. Dwyer FC. Osteotomy of the calcaneum for pes cavus. J Bone Joint Surg Br 1959;41:80–6.
11. Myerson MS, Kadakia AR. Reconstructive foot and ankle surgery: management of complications E-Book. Philadelphia: Elsevier Health Sciences; 2018.
12. VanValkenburg S, Hsu RY, Palmer DS, et al. Neurologic deficit associated with lateralizing calcaneal osteotomy for cavovarus foot correction. Foot Ankle Int 2016; 37:1106–12.

An Approach to Managing Midfoot Charcot Deformities

Ashtin Doorgakant, MBBS, FRCS (Tr & Orth)[a],*, Mark B. Davies, BM, FRCS, FRCS (Tr & Orth)[b]

KEYWORDS

- Diabetes • Charcot neuroarthropathy • Midfoot • Deformity • Deformity correction

KEY POINTS

- Charcot neuroarthropathy and its complications are on the rise as incidence of diabetes keeps increasing worldwide.
- Emphasis is on prevention and early detection via a well-run surveillance program with clear guidelines.
- Mainstay of initial management remains nonoperative within a multidisciplinary team.
- Surgical treatment of Charcot neuroarthropathy is evolving with more evidence for early intervention and usage of "superconstructs," especially in grossly unstable situations.
- There is a role for debridement, exostectomy, and Achilles tendon lengthening on their own or as adjunctive procedures.

 Video content accompanies this article at http://www.foot.theclinics.com.

BACKGROUND

Charcot neuroarthropathy (CN) is a debilitating condition associated with peripheral neuropathy, which can result in severe deformities, primarily in the foot and ankle.[1] Today, it mostly affects patients with diabetes[2] but it can be secondary to any cause of neuropathy.

The incidence of CN was reported at 0.3/1000 per year in 2000[3] but is increasing with a corresponding rise in incidence of diabetes. According to the National Institute for Health and Care Excellence (NICE), the prevalence of diabetes in the United Kingdom has gone from 1.9 million in 2006 to 2.9 million in 2013 and is expected to rise to 5.0 million in 2025.[4] A similar picture is seen worldwide with an estimated 450 million diabetic patients in 2015, expected to reach 642 million by 2040.[5,6]

Diabetic complications are not benign. Many studies have reported a 5-year mortality rate, as high as 50%, after first-time diabetic ulceration.[7] A similar prognosis is true

[a] Foot and Ankle Unit, Northern General Hospital, Foot and Ankle Offices, Selby Wing, Herries Road, Sheffield S5 7AU, UK; [b] Northern General Hospital, Foot and Ankle Unit, Herries Road, Sheffield, S5 7AU, UK
* Corresponding author.
E-mail address: ashtindoorgakant@yahoo.co.uk

Foot Ankle Clin N Am 25 (2020) 319–335
https://doi.org/10.1016/j.fcl.2020.02.009
foot.theclinics.com
1083-7515/20/Crown Copyright © 2020 Published by Elsevier Inc. All rights reserved.

for diabetic-related amputations.[8] The exact mortality rate following CN is not clearly reported in the literature but is likely to be high. Mortality and amputation risks are less than those of diabetic ulceration in the absence of CN,[6] possibly because of the increased vascularity in CN feet.[9] Wukich and colleagues[10] found that even though CN can coexist with peripheral vascular disease, this is much less than for non-Charcot diabetic feet (odds ratio 0.48). It is often suggested that peripheral vascular disease, and by inference old age, are somewhat protective against CN but not against diabetic ulceration. Indeed, the typical patient with CN is an obese patient in their mid-50s who has been diabetic for at least 10 years.[11]

PATHOPHYSIOLOGY

The exact pathophysiology of CN is not fully understood. Peripheral neuropathy needs to be present first and the pathophysiology of this also has not been fully described.[12] It is certainly multifactorial with several proposed mechanisms.[13] Irrespective of the type of diabetes, cumulative poor glycemic control has been shown to be the single most important factor in initiating the development and progression of neuropathy.[13,14]

Peripheral neuropathy can affect sensory, motor, and/or autonomic function. Often all 3 modalities are involved, resulting in repetitive microtraumatic and microvascular insults. Each deficit contributes to the pathogenesis of CN in a different way. Sensory neuropathy removes the protective sensation and proprioception of normal feet. Thus, automatic reactions, such as guarding, weight-shifting, and activity limitation are lost.[15] Motor neuropathy can cause muscle wasting in an unbalanced way. Weakness of the anterior and lateral leg compartments can lead to claw toe and equinus ankle deformities, respectively.[16] This, in turn, increases forefoot and midfoot plantar pressures, predisposing to ulceration and midfoot collapse. Autonomic neuropathy leads to sudomotor abnormalities, resulting in dry easily-cracked skin and more importantly in sympathetic denervation. This causes arteriovenous shunting diverting blood away from the skin, producing a warmer foot than normal.[13]

The prevalence of CN in patients with peripheral neuropathy is only 0.09% to 1.4%.[17] Therefore, the progression to CN likely involves other trigger factors. There is typically an inflammation-producing event preceding the development of an acute Charcot process. This event may be a sprain, an infection, fracture, or surgery to the foot and ankle. The underlying pathophysiological process that triggers the acute CN is thought to be a hyperemic response that does not switch off spontaneously.[18] There is a sudden increase in blood flow, bringing with it a surge of proinflammatory cytokines.[12] Receptor activator of nuclear factor-kB ligand (RANKL) is also upregulated, resulting in an elevated RANKL to osteoprotegerin ratio. Osteoclastic activity surpasses osteoblastic activity, accelerating bone resorption. RANKL is also responsible for the calcification of arteries, seen radiographically in up to 90% of patients with CN[19] (**Fig. 1**).

CLASSIFICATION AND ASSESSMENT

Earlier stages of CN are difficult to distinguish from differentials such as infection, gout, deep venous thrombosis, and minor trauma. As the condition progresses, deformities develop and give rise to problems with footwear and risk of ulceration. The progression has been described by Eichenholtz into stages 1 to 3 based on clinical and radiographic findings[20] (**Table 1**). A stage 0 was subsequently added by Shibata and colleagues in 1990[21] to describe an inflamed foot without any radiographic changes of CN. An alternate stage 0 has been described by Yu and Hudson[22] to describe a clinically quiescent foot at risk of CN. Chantelau and Poll[23] showed that MRI changes are already apparent in stage 0.

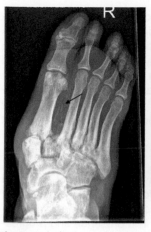
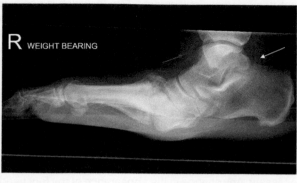

Fig. 1. Calcified vessels (*arrows*) typically attributed to elevated RANKL activity in Charcot.

The distribution of CN is also important. This has been classified by Sanders and Frykberg[24] and later modified by Brodsky (**Table 2** and **3**).[25]

Further attempts at classifying CN specific to the midfoot have been made. In 1998, Sammarco and Conti[26] described 5 typical patterns of dislocation and/or collapse.

Table 1

Eichenholtz classification with modifications by Shibata and colleagues[21] and Yu and Hudson[22]

Stage	Description	Clinical Features	Imaging
0 (Shibata) 0 (Yu, Hudson)	The "at-risk" foot	Inflamed foot Neuropathic foot with trauma	Radiographs: normal. MRI: bone edema, stress fractures, soft tissue edema, joint effusion.
1	Fragmentation (acute phase)	Warmth (>2°C c/f unaffected side), erythema, swelling. Onset of deformity.	Radiographs: Disorganization of joints with bone debris, subchondral fragmentation, periarticular fractures, subluxations, and dislocations. Osteopenia.
2	Coalescence (subacute phase)	Reduced warmth (<2°C c/f unaffected side), erythema and swelling. Progression or maintenance of deformity.	Radiographs: Fine debris resorption, new callus formation, coalescence of fractures, periarticular sclerosis.
3	Consolidation (chronic phase)	Resolution of warmth, erythema and swelling. Consolidation of deformity.	Radiographs: Consolidation of fractures and remodeling of bones. Reduction of sclerosis.

c/f, compared with.

Data from Trepman E, Nihal A, Pinzur MS. Current topics review: Charcot neuroarthropathy of the foot and ankle. *Foot Ankle Int.* 2005;26(1):46-63 and Miller RJ. Neuropathic Minimally Invasive Surgeries (NEMESIS):: Percutaneous Diabetic Foot Surgery and Reconstruction. *Foot Ankle Clin.* 2016;21(3):595-627.

This included a new radiographic measure of midfoot dislocation, the so-called "bayonet-type" dorsal displacement (**Fig. 2**), which is poorly identified by both anteroposterior (AP) and lateral talo-first-metatarsal angle or talonavicular coverage angle. Schon and colleagues[27] later suggested a classification system comprising 4 distinct anatomic patterns and an extra stage for severity, the Beta stage. Their study aimed to better define the apex of the deformity and predict who was at higher risk of poor clinical outcome and had good inter/intraobserver reliability.[28] Both systems appeared independent of the Eichenholtz staging but neither offered systematic management algorithms.

Clinical Assessment

The treating physician or surgeon needs to be able to assess the Charcot foot at all stages. In all diabetic patients, a regular screening and foot protection program are necessary. Any change in the appearance of the foot needs to be considered with suspicion, and foot protection escalated if any doubt exists. The presence and progression of any ulcer needs to be meticulously documented. A probe to bone test is highly suggestive of concomitant osteomyelitis.[29] Sensory examination is best done with a Semmes-Weinstein 5.07 monofilament.[30] Equinus and/or claw toe deformities should be identified and a Silfverskiold test undertaken.

Stage 1 can mimic an infective process, especially in the presence of a diabetic ulcer. Indeed, the 2 can present concomitantly. Clinical assessment will reveal swelling, erythema, and a warm foot at least 2°C higher than the unaffected side. One test that sometimes favors a diagnosis of CN is a decrease in erythema after foot elevation. Lack of general malaise and blood sugar derangement seen in sepsis also point toward CN.[16]

Stage 2 begins once the foot swelling, erythema, and warmth start to decrease with the skin temperature difference between feet returning to less than 2°C.[31] The foot is still potentially unstable at this stage and further deformation may occur. Further callus formation may accentuate any bony prominences from deformity.

Conventionally, Stage 3 was considered the "safe" stage to initiate surgical correction of the foot, because bony consolidation occurs with resolution of significant inflammation. Full remodeling may not be complete until months later.[20]

Radiological Assessment

One of the problems with CN is that there are no definitive clinical or laboratory diagnostic criteria making mild or early cases difficult to distinguish from osteomyelitis.[32]

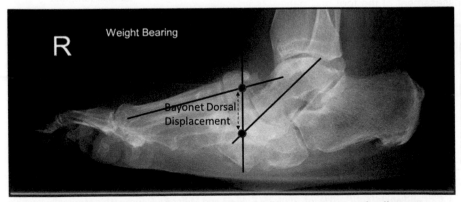

Fig. 2. Bayonet-type dorsal displacement as described by Sammarco and colleagues.

Advances in the field of imaging have made these distinctions more reliable. Osteopenia is commonly seen at all stages.[4] On plain standing AP and lateral radiographs, deformity, collapse and bony prominences are easily recognizable. Radiographic parameters used in grading severity and planning deformity correction are listed in **Table 4**.

Computed tomography (CT) scanning is of limited diagnostic value and is mainly used to assist surgical planning.[33] In this case, a 3-dimensional (3D) model can be a useful tool (**Fig. 3**). However, with the use of standing CT becoming more widespread, this may supersede plain radiography as a monitor of disease progression, and still assist in surgical planning. MRI scans have a high sensitivity (77%–100%) and specificity (80%–100%) for osteomyelitis, but the specificity against CN is less, especially in chronic stages. Ledermann and Morrison[34] suggested a combined approach in which clinical signs are considered. The presence of ulcers, sinus tracts, fluid collections, and certain anatomic distribution patterns are more suggestive of osteomyelitis.[34] Nuclear medicine modalities like white-cell–labeled technetium (99mTc HMPAO) and PET-CT can yield even greater sensitivities and specificities.[35] However, access to these modalities is limited and expensive and cannot be advocated for widespread use.

NONOPERATIVE MANAGEMENT

Morbidity from CN is significant and early recognition and treatment is essential in limiting the damage. The aim of treatment is the "achievement of an ulcer and infection-free plantigrade foot that can be managed longitudinally with simple commercially available therapeutic footwear."[36]

Most Charcot feet are initially managed nonoperatively. Management of CN starts with a foot surveillance program allowing for early identification of problems. In the United Kingdom, there are very clear guidelines for diabetic foot management generated by both NICE and the British Orthopedic Association.[4] These guidelines emphasize the need for patient education, foot screening clinics, and a multidisciplinary foot protection service. The latter is usually led by a diabetologist who ensures optimal diabetic control and monitoring of HbA1c. A review of the literature by Smith and colleagues[37] on the impact of nonsurgical interventions for CN concluded that bisphosphonates may improve the healing of Charcot foot by reducing skin temperature and disease activity of the Charcot foot, when applied in addition to standard interventions to control the position and shape of the foot. Podiatrists help with assessment of the foot and paring down calluses and, together with orthotists, can

Table 2
Sanders and Frykberg anatomic classification[24]

Type	Location	Frequency, %
1	Forefoot	15
2	Tarsometatarsal joint	40
3a	Naviculo-cuneiform/Talonavicular/Calcaneocuboid joints	30
3b	Ankle/Subtalar joints	10
4	Calcaneus	5

Data from Sanders LJ, Frykberg RG. Diabetic neuropathic osteoarthropathy: the Charcot foot. In:- Frykberg RG, editor. The high risk foot in diabetes mellitus. New York: Churchill Livingstone; 1991:297–338.

Table 3 Brodsky[25] anatomic classification		
Type	Location	Frequency, %
1	Tarsometatarsal/Naviculo-cuneiform joints	60
2	Talonavicular/Calcaneocuboid/Subtalar joints	10
3a	Tibiotalar joint	20
3b	Calcaneal tuberosity	<10
4	Combination of areas	<10
5	Forefoot	<10

Data from Trepman E, Nihal A, Pinzur MS. Current topics review: Charcot neuroarthropathy of the foot and ankle. *Foot Ankle Int.* 2005;26(1):46-63 and Miller RJ. Neuropathic Minimally Invasive Surgeries (NEMESIS):: Percutaneous Diabetic Foot Surgery and Reconstruction. *Foot Ankle Clin.* 2016;21(3):595-627.

decide on the appropriate form of foot protection. This can be in the form of molded insoles, bespoke shoes, braces, or total contact casting. Input from specially trained plaster technicians and dedicated orthotists is essential for appropriate customized casting and brace fitting, such as the Charcot Restraint Orthotic Walkers (CROW).[38] Suitable orthotics can obviate the need for surgery in up to half of patients with CN.[39]

In the acute phase (Eichenholtz 1) of CN, the foot may or may not already be deformed. Unless there is a deformity that would preclude containment of the foot in a brace or plaster and cause inevitable ulceration, a total contact cast (TCC) is recommended **(Fig. 4)**.[40] The TCC helps distribute pressure throughout the foot with minimal focal peak pressures. Subtle variations in design exist, for example, fully closed or "open-toe" models. Casts need changing every 1 to 2 weeks for up to 18 weeks or more until the foot has progressed into stage 2. If an ulcer is already present, the TCC also will help with ulcer healing, especially for Wagner grades 1 and 2.[41] Antibiotics may be required if there is concomitant infection. The most reliable method of isolating the causative organism is through a bone biopsy.[42] Prevention of weight bearing is essential in this period to rest the soft tissues and avoid any further changes to the midfoot architecture. This can be assisted with the application of a Bohler stirrup to transfer weight more proximally to the shin. Once the patient has reached stage 2, a removable brace with a molded total contact insole or CROW boot may be used. Sometimes the patient is unable to comply with a cast and/or non–weight-bearing instructions, and a more pragmatic approach with a brace, partial weight bearing, or a wheelchair and close supervision may be required. If possible, weight bearing should be initiated only once the foot is stable (Video 1).

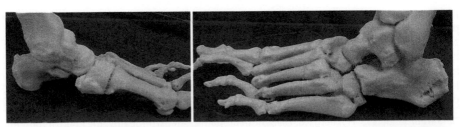

Fig. 3. Three-dimensional CT model. This can be used to identify clearly where the deformity lies for resection planning and deciding about hardware options.

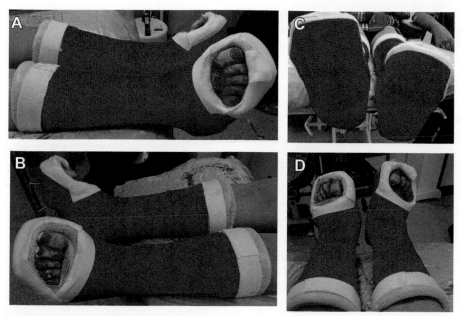

Fig. 4. An example of a total contact cast. (*A*) Right side view. (*B*) End view. (*C*) Left side view. (*D*) Top view.

SURGICAL MANAGEMENT

Surgical correction of deformity is indicated to prevent complications from CN. Unless in the presence of clinical urgency within stage 1, it was conventional that deformity surgery would be undertaken in late stage 2 or stage 3. Typical indications for surgery include the following:

- A high risk of ulceration from deformity
- Established osteomyelitis, resistant to antibiotics
- Inability to prevent weight bearing and/or inadequate bracing in an unstable foot[15]

This convention is being challenged with more contemporary studies describing earlier surgical intervention during stage 1 to limit development of the deformity before correction.[43,44]

The aim of surgery in CN of the midfoot is to restore a stable painless plantigrade and infection-free foot that can be fitted with bespoke footwear with minimal risk of ulceration. Sometimes that is not possible, and a higher-level amputation is the only remaining option. Local surgery can take the form of a debridement, exostectomy, osteotomy, fusion, limited amputation, or more commonly a combination of these techniques.[45] Frequently, a concomitant Tendo Achilles or gastrocnemius lengthening is necessary if there is any evidence of hindfoot equinus. Adequate vascular supply is a prerequisite for orthopedic foot surgery, necessitating input from vascular specialists. In the presence of complex wounds and ulceration that preclude a primary closure or application of topical negative pressure therapy, the expertise of a plastic surgeon also may be necessary. Wound healing can be a real issue in the diabetic foot and the recently developed concept of angiosomes will assist the surgeon in placing their incisions in the most favorable way.[46]

Midfoot deformities typically appear as a collapse of the medial and lateral longitudinal arches and are commonly associated with coronal plane deformities of the forefoot and hindfoot, namely abduction and valgus. The deformity occurs along a spectrum, the end stage of which is a rocker bottom deformity with midfoot dislocation. Sometimes single areas of acute deformity or bony prominence from callus or dislocations can become a threat to the skin.

Careful surgical planning is mandated for a successful outcome. The following variables play a key role in deciding the optimal surgical strategy:

- Patient compliance
- Severity of deformity
- Apex of deformity
- Soft tissue quality
- Bone quality
- Bone loss
- Vascular status
- Eichenholtz stage
- Ulceration
- Osteomyelitis
- Patient preference
- Medical comorbidities

There are no studies to compare one surgical modality against another and this is complicated further because most procedures involve a combination of different surgical techniques. Furthermore, publications on individual methods tend to be results of case series (Level IV evidence) or expert opinions (Level V evidence). Lowery and colleagues[47] conducted a thorough review of the literature in 2012 and found that there was inconclusive evidence for surgery in Eichenholtz stage 1 despite some encouraging results (2 studies[48,49]) nor was there any advantage of one form of internal fixation over another.

Interestingly, a further systematic review undertaken by Shazadeh Safavi and colleagues[44] in 2017 identified 5 more contemporary studies in which surgery was recommended for stage 1 with acceptable results. Their primary outcome measure were the rates of transtibial amputation and midfoot fusion rates. These were found to be 6% and 91%, respectively, indicating an overall good result from surgery. More recently, Kroin and colleagues[50] demonstrated a significant improvement in quality of life of surgery versus immobilization in early stages of CN.

Debridement

Diabetic ulcers initially should be treated nonoperatively, as previously described. Recalcitrant ulcers and deep soft tissue infections raise the possibility of osteomyelitis and are best managed with surgical debridement.[51] The surgical approach needs to be carefully planned to try to achieve primary closure.[52] Sometimes primary wound closure may not be achievable and topical negative pressure therapy may be adequate, especially in the presence of small wounds. Larger soft tissue defects may require the input of a plastic surgeon.[45]

In established osteomyelitis, treatment is by debridement to healthy bleeding bone, guided by preoperative MRI and intraoperative visualization. Deep tissue samples are sent for microbiology and histology. Antibiotic-laden cement or antibiotic-loaded biocomposites, such as calcium sulfate and hydroxyapatite compounds, can be added to deep bony surfaces to enhance local infection clearance.[53,54] There also may be a role in applying some biocomposites into the surrounding soft tissue envelope. Jogia and colleagues[55] presented a series of 20 patients treated with gentamicin-impregnated and vancomycin-impregnated calcium sulfate pellets inserted into fenestrations within the medullary cavity of debrided bone. They report complete wound healing at a median of 5 weeks and no recurrence of osteomyelitis within 12 months. A 2-stage procedure is preferred by some surgeons, with the first stage aimed at controlling the infection, with temporary fixation away from the septic zone in the form of buried wires[56] or an external fixator or frame. The second stage of definitive fixation goes ahead once wounds have healed and inflammatory markers have settled.

Exostectomy

In the presence of a bony prominence abnormally loading the soft tissue envelope threatening or causing ulceration, then removal of prominent bone alone may suffice (**Fig. 5**).[57] Catanzariti and colleagues[58] found a higher risk of complications and recurrence with laterally based prominences due to rotation of the cuboid. The prominence can be removed via a direct open incision with the aim of disseminating the pressure of bearing weight across a smooth surface. More recently, minimally invasive approaches have been used with the purported advantage of avoiding a plantar wound, reducing the risk of infection.[59]

Osteotomy and Fusion

When the midfoot is grossly deformed and/or unstable, surgical correction may be required. Small deformity correction can be achieved by fusing involved joints in situ with minimal bone resection. Larger corrections may require osteotomies planned at the apex of the deformity. The deformity may be multiplanar, requiring more complex planning of incisions and osteotomies. Closing wedge osteotomies have the advantage of shortening the foot, thereby alleviating tension on the soft tissues and facilitating wound closure. Conversely, opening wedge osteotomies often require bone graft and may compromise closure of the soft tissue envelope, have the potential to collapse, and can act as a medium for infection.[60,61] Conventionally,

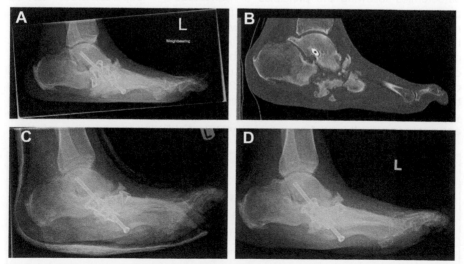

Fig. 5. (A) Preoperative radiograph showing residual plantar prominence associated with ulceration following previous surgery for CN. (B) Preoperative CT. (C) Post-MIS resection radiograph (2 weeks). (D) Postoperative radiograph (6 weeks) fully healed ulcer.

osteotomies have been through open incisions. Jones[62] describes a biplanar osteotomy for the rocker bottom foot, which removes a medial and plantar closing wedge (apex dorsolateral), through which rotation can also be dialed. When no midfoot dislocation is present, an all-medial approach is advocated by some researchers.[63] By using curved osteotomes, a lateral hinge is preserved at the level of the cuboid, which acts as a tension band once the osteotomy is closed and fixed medially, thereby avoiding a second incision laterally. This avoids violating the lateral angiosome, whose vascularity is more tenuous.[46] More recent studies have hailed the benefit of percutaneous osteotomies using osteotomes or burrs.[6] The advocates of these minimally invasive procedures often use fine wire circular fixators or percutaneous screw fixation techniques.[64]

Sammarco[41] expounded the concept of "superconstructs" in stabilizing the grossly unstable foot following osteotomy, owing to the high risk of hardware failure in short-segment stabilization. Superconstructs are defined by 4 factors (**Box 1, Fig. 6, Table 4**).

Methods of stabilization include plates, intramedullary beams, and circular frames. The presence of infection precludes placement of internal hardware and is a relative indication for fine wire external fixation or to consider a staged approach once infection has been eradicated.[41] The presence of ulcers, even when not infected, also must be considered a relative contraindication for internal fixation. Ford and colleagues[68] highlighted an increased infection risk and amputation rate when applying internal fixation techniques in the presence of ulceration.

External Fixation

Circular frame fixation allows for placement of pins away from ulcers, poor-quality skin, and potentially infected bone. Infected bone that has been debrided and treated with appropriate antibiotics is still not suitable for internal metalwork application but can heal satisfactorily when stabilized externally, even as a single-stage procedure.[69] In patients with no evidence of infection or compromise to the soft tissue envelope, osteotomies following the principles of Sammarco's[41] "superconstruct" can be planned by assessing the deformity in all 3 planes. Preoperative planning with simulation software or on a 3D model may improve the planning process for frame application. A neutral ring fixator can be applied in situ with compression after appropriate debridement and realignment. This can be preassembled as a static 3-level ring construct made of a foot plate and 2 tibial rings connected to the bone via tensioned olive wires. Pinzur[64] reports a series of 26 patients with significant comorbidities treated with that technique, and 24 of them were infection-free and ulcer-free at a year. An alternative way of correcting the deformity is by performing an osteotomy and applying a "butt frame" such as a Taylor Spatial Frame to mirror the deformity,

---

Box 1
"Superconstruct" defining criteria

Fusion beyond the osteotomy to include unaffected joints strengthens the fixation

Bone resection shortens the foot and reduces soft tissue tension

Use of the strongest device tolerated by the soft tissues

Application of devices in a position that maximizes mechanical function

Data from Sammarco VJ. Superconstructs in the treatment of charcot foot deformity: plantar plating, locked plating, and axial screw fixation. *Foot Ankle Clin.* 2009;14(3):393-407.

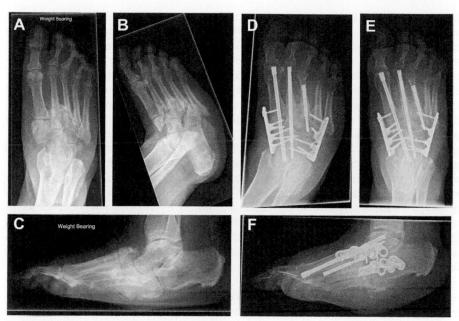

Fig. 6. "Superconstruct" principles. (*A–C*) Preoperative radiographs of severe rocker-bottom deformity: Eichenholtz stage 3. (*D–F*) Postoperative imaging of middle, central and lateral column fixation using intramuscular beams and locking plates after closing wedge osteotomy.

and then dialing in the correction via a software.[70] Because the pin sites can act as stress risers in osteopenic bone, bearing weight through the frame is usually not allowed in the first month. Once the osteotomy has healed, protection for a further 4 to 6 weeks in a total contact cast or other orthotic is continued, permitting weight bearing.

Internal Fixation

Plates

The use of plates has been greatly enhanced with the advent of locking technology. Locked plates with fixed angle screws provide improved fixation in osteoporotic

Table 4			
Useful radiographic measurements in defining midfoot Charcot neuroarthropathy deformity			
Measurement	**Angle/ Line**	**View**	**Normal Value**
Talus: first metatarsal	Angle	AP	7° (3–11)
Talus: first metatarsal (Meary)	Angle	Lateral	6° (2–10)
Talo-navicular coverage angle	Angle	AP	<7°
Calcaneal: fifth metatarsal	Angle	Lateral	150°–170°
Calcaneal pitch	Angle	Lateral	18° (13–23)
Cuboid (lateral column) height	Line	Lateral	12 mm (8–16)

Abbreviation: AP, anteroposterior
Data from Refs.[65–67]

bone, effectively acting as "internal fixators."[71] Nonlocking plates also can be used in varying modes of application with intrinsic or extrinsic compression, but when applied on the plantar aspect of the midfoot, they can be used in tension-band mode. Despite the increasing popularity of locking plates, meaningful studies documenting results following their use are sparse. Observing Sammarco's[41] superconstruct principles, multiple plates may need to be applied across the columns of the foot. Medial and dorsal approaches can be used to apply plates, with a more plantar incision for applying a plantar plate in tension-band mode. Applying plates on the tension side of the foot is biomechanically superior and enhances compression during weight bearing.[72,73] An additional perceived advantage is that plates applied to the plantar aspect of the foot are well covered by soft tissues but, paradoxically, gaining good surgical access to apply them can be tricky. Schon and colleagues[74] used plantar plating in 34 of 131 patients with midfoot Charcot and achieved a satisfactory level of correction and fusion. Even though they did not separate 3 patients who had frame correction from the 37 who required surgery following failed conservative management of midfoot CN, there were only 7 minor reoperations and 90% of patients were satisfied, with all but 1 returning to regular or orthopedic footwear.

Intramedullary beam (axial screw fixation)

Inserting a long, cannulated, wide-bore intramedullary screw or bolt acting as a beam along 1 or more columns of the foot has gained popularity. In the presence of a minor deformity, simple preparation of the joints to be spanned by the beam for fusion may suffice. However, in more significant deformity, osteotomies are necessary to achieve adequate correction before stabilizing with a columnar beam. Insertion of a beam to the medial column is through the first metatarsophalangeal joint (MTPJ) with the beam applied into the talus. Smaller-diameter beams can be applied through the second and third MTPJs. Beams applied to the lateral column gain proximal hold in the calcaneus. Through open approaches, access to the columns can be achieved though the osteotomy or joint, allowing the beam guidewire to be applied in both a retrograde and antegrade manner along the column. The screw is recessed quite deeply after insertion to preserve MTPJ motion. Beam fixation can then be further augmented with plates or a frame if required. Ford and colleagues[68] report on 25 cases with satisfactory AP and lateral Meary angle corrections in an ulcer-free foot in 84% of patients. However at 18 months, fewer than half of the osteotomies had united (46%), with almost 20% requiring proximal amputation, especially in those patients with preexisting ulcers. Eschler and colleagues[75] observed a 42% amputation rate and a 29% rate of bony union with beam fixation of the median column alone. They recommend combining it with another stabilization procedure, such as plating. Sammarco and colleagues[76] had better union rates in their series of 22 patients using beams alone, with 16 unions at 6 months. All their patients returned to independent functional ambulation at 10 months.

Introduction of column beams using minimally invasive techniques has been advocated and given the acronym NEMISIS (neuropathic minimally invasive surgery). With minimal disruption of the soft tissue envelope, the bony cuts are made with a 20-mm Shannon burr, guided by pre-placed 2-mm Kirschner wires and the wedge of bone to be resected is made into a paste that is then squeezed out before the intramuscular beams are inserted as discussed.[6] With the 16 patients treated in this manner, Miller[77] observed a 25% deep infection rate and half of the patients required further surgery, including metalwork removals, revision fixation, and exostectomy. However, no patients proceeded to major amputation.

Hindfoot equinus deformity correction

Multiple procedures exist for correcting hindfoot equinus. Lengthening of the Achilles tendon can be performed in isolation or as an ancillary procedure to bony or other soft tissue corrections. Hastings and colleagues[78] demonstrated a reduction in peak plantar pressures following lengthening. This has been partly attributed to relief of the contracture and partly to weakened plantarflexion.[47,78] Performing the Strayer or Baumann's procedure addresses isolated gastrocnemius tightness, but if the whole triceps surae is tight, the Hoke percutaneous triple hemi-section of the Achilles tendon is very effective.[79] In very severe contractures, a formal Z-lengthening of the Tendo Achilles may be required. As a final word of caution, if the calcaneal pitch is already elevated, such as in a cavovarus foot, a tendon-lengthening procedure in the absence of a true contracture could worsen the problem.[80]

SUMMARY

The treatment of midfoot deformities associated with CN remains one of the most complex problems facing the orthopedic foot and ankle surgeon. The heterogeneity of presentation means that meaningful large-number studies comparing different modes of treatment are difficult to achieve. The best evidence remains at level 4 and new approaches are being introduced based on biomechanical theories rather than well-conducted trials. Nonetheless, there appears to be a gradual refinement in the overall outcome. With diabetes reaching epidemic proportions, it is likely that we will be seeing more of these cases. Therefore, a more robust algorithm to managing CN of the foot and ankle will need to be developed. Right now, a high degree of vigilance to improve early detection of the condition, along with a carefully planned multidisciplinary approach to treatment, in which outcomes of interventions including surgery are carefully monitored, offers our best hope to one day getting the better of this problem. An emphasis on prevention and optimal diabetic control should be the central tenets of this approach.

DISCLOSURE

The authors have nothing to disclose.

SUPPLEMENTARY DATA

Supplementary data related to this article can be found online at https://doi.org/10.1016/j.fcl.2020.02.009.

REFERENCES

1. Sinha S, Munichoodappa CS, Kozak GP. Neuro-arthropathy (Charcot joints) in diabetes mellitus. Medicine 1972;51(3):191–210.
2. Rogers LC, Frykberg RG, Armstrong DG, et al. The Charcot foot in diabetes. Diabetes Care 2011;34(9):2123–9.
3. Fabrin J, Larsen K, Holstein PE. Long-term follow-up in diabetic Charcot feet with spontaneous onset. Diabetes Care 2000;23(6):796–800.
4. National Institute for Health and Clinical Excellence. Diabetic foot problems: prevention and management. NICE guidelines [NG19]. 2015.
5. Ibrahim A. IDF clinical practice recommendation on the diabetic foot: a guide for healthcare professionals. Diabetes Res Clin Pract 2017;127:285–7.
6. Miller RJ. Neuropathic minimally invasive surgeries (NEMESIS): percutaneous diabetic foot surgery and reconstruction. Foot Ankle Clin 2016;21(3):595–627.

7. Moulik PK, Mtonga R, Gill GV. Amputation and mortality in new-onset diabetic foot ulcers stratified by etiology. Diabetes Care 2003;26(2):491–4.

8. Armstrong DG, Wrobel J, Robbins JM. Guest Editorial: are diabetes-related wounds and amputations worse than cancer? Int Wound J 2007;4(4):286–7.

9. Sohn MW, Stuck RM, Pinzur M, et al. Lower-extremity amputation risk after charcot arthropathy and diabetic foot ulcer. Diabetes Care 2010;33(1):98–100.

10. Wukich DK, Raspovic KM, Suder NC. Prevalence of peripheral arterial disease in patients with diabetic charcot neuroarthropathy. J Foot Ankle Surg 2016;55(4): 727–31.

11. Game FL, Catlow R, Jones GR, et al. Audit of acute Charcot's disease in the UK: the CDUK study. Diabetologia 2012;55(1):32–5.

12. Jeffcoate W. The causes of the Charcot syndrome. Clin Podiatr Med Surg 2008; 25(1):29–42, vi.

13. Bibbo C, Patel DV. Diabetic neuropathy. Foot Ankle Clin 2006;11(4):753–74.

14. Nathan DM, Genuth S, Lachin J, et al. The effect of intensive treatment of diabetes on the development and progression of long-term complications in insulin-dependent diabetes mellitus. N Engl J Med 1993;329(14):977–86.

15. Trepman E, Nihal A, Pinzur MS. Current topics review: Charcot neuroarthropathy of the foot and ankle. Foot Ankle Int 2005;26(1):46–63.

16. Pinzur MS. An evidence-based introduction to charcot foot arthropathy. Foot & Ankle Orthopaedics 2018;3(3). 2473011418774269.

17. Frykberg RG, Belczyk R. Epidemiology of the Charcot foot. Clin Podiatr Med Surg 2008;25(1):17–28, v.

18. Christensen TM, Simonsen L, Holstein PE, et al. Sympathetic neuropathy in diabetes mellitus patients does not elicit Charcot osteoarthropathy. J Diabetes Complications 2011;25(5):320–4.

19. Clouse ME, Gramm HF, Legg M, et al. Diabetic osteoarthropathy. Clinical and roentgenographic observations in 90 cases. Am J Roentgenol Radium Ther Nucl Med 1974;121(1):22–34.

20. Eichenholtz SN. Charcot Joints. [S.l.]: Thomas; 1966.

21. Shibata T, Tada K, Hashizume C. The results of arthrodesis of the ankle for leprotic neuroarthropathy. J Bone Joint Surg Am 1990;72(5):749–56.

22. Yu GV, Hudson JR. Evaluation and treatment of stage 0 Charcot's neuroarthropathy of the foot and ankle. J Am Podiatr Med Assoc 2002;92(4):210–20.

23. Chantelau E, Poll LW. Evaluation of the diabetic charcot foot by MR imaging or plain radiography–an observational study. Exp Clin Endocrinol Diabetes 2006; 114(8):428–31.

24. Sanders L, Frykberg R. Diabetic neuropathic osteoarthropathy: the Charcot foot. In: Frykberg RG, editor. The high risk foot in diabetes mellitus. New York: Churchill Livingstone; 1991.

25. Coughlin M, Saltzman C, Anderson RA, editors. Surgery of the foot and ankle. 9th edition. London: Mosby; 2013.

26. Sammarco GJ, Conti SF. Surgical treatment of neuroarthropathic foot deformity. Foot Ankle Int 1998;19(2):102–9.

27. Schon LC, Weinfeld SB, Horton GA, et al. Radiographic and clinical classification of acquired midtarsus deformities. Foot Ankle Int 1998;19(6):394–404.

28. Schon LC, Easley ME, Cohen I, et al. The acquired midtarsus deformity classification system–interobserver reliability and intraobserver reproducibility. Foot Ankle Int 2002;23(1):30–6.

29. Grayson ML, Gibbons GW, Balogh K, et al. Probing to bone in infected pedal ulcers: a clinical sign of underlying osteomyelitis in diabetic patients. JAMA 1995; 273(9):721–3.
30. Tanenberg R, Schumer M, Greene D, et al. Neuropathic problems of the lower extremities in diabetic patients. In: Bowker JH, Pfeifer MA, editors. Levin and O'Neal's the diabetic foot. 6th edition. London: Mosby; 2001. with forewords by Paul W. Brand, Gary W. Gibbons, Fred W. Whitehouse.
31. Papanas N, Maltezos E. Etiology, pathophysiology and classifications of the diabetic Charcot foot. Diabet Foot Ankle 2013;4. https://doi.org/10.3402/dfa.v4i0.20872.
32. Yousaf S, Dawe EJC, Saleh A, et al. The acute Charcot foot in diabetics: diagnosis and management. EFORT Open Rev 2018;3(10):568–73.
33. Rogers LC, Bevilacqua NJ. Imaging of the Charcot foot. Clin Podiatr Med Surg 2008;25(2):263–74, vii.
34. Ledermann HP, Morrison WB. Differential diagnosis of pedal osteomyelitis and diabetic neuroarthropathy: MR imaging. Semin Musculoskelet Radiol 2005;9(3): 272–83.
35. Peterson N, Widnall J, Evans P, et al. Diagnostic imaging of diabetic foot disorders. Foot Ankle Int 2017;38(1):86–95.
36. Harkln EA, Schneider AM, Murphy M, et al. Deformity and clinical outcomes following operative correction of charcot ankle. Foot Ankle Int 2019;40(2):145–51.
37. Smith C, Kumar S, Causby R. The effectiveness of non-surgical interventions in the treatment of Charcot foot. Int J Evid Based Healthc 2007;5(4):437–49.
38. Mehta JA, Brown C, Sargeant N. Charcot restraint orthotic walker. Foot Ankle Int 1998;19(9):619–23.
39. Pinzur M. Surgical versus accommodative treatment for Charcot arthropathy of the midfoot. Foot Ankle Int 2004;25(8):545–9.
40. Jostel A, Jude EB. Medical treatment of Charcot neuroosteoarthropathy. Clin Podiatr Med Surg 2008;25(1):63–9, vi-vii.
41. Sammarco VJ. Superconstructs in the treatment of charcot foot deformity: plantar plating, locked plating, and axial screw fixation. Foot Ankle Clin 2009;14(3): 393–407.
42. Ertugrul BM, Lipsky BA, Savk O. Osteomyelitis or Charcot neuroosteoarthropathy? Differentiating these disorders in diabetic patients with a foot problem. Diabet Foot Ankle 2013;4. https://doi.org/10.3402/dfa.v4i0.21855.
43. Wukich DK, Sung W. Charcot arthropathy of the foot and ankle: modern concepts and management review. J Diabetes Complications 2009;23(6):409–26.
44. Shazadeh Safavi P, Jupiter DC, Panchbhavi V. A systematic review of current surgical interventions for charcot neuroarthropathy of the midfoot. J Foot Ankle Surg 2017;56(6):1249–52.
45. Sponer P, Kucera T, Brtkova J, et al. The management of Charcot midfoot deformities in diabetic patients. Acta Medica (Hradec Kralove) 2013;56(1):3–8.
46. Clemens MW, Attinger CE. Angiosomes and wound care in the diabetic foot. Foot Ankle Clin 2010;15(3):439–64.
47. Lowery NJ, Woods JB, Armstrong DG, et al. Surgical management of Charcot neuroarthropathy of the foot and ankle: a systematic review. Foot Ankle Int 2012;33(2):113–21.
48. Simon SR, Tejwani SG, Wilson DL, et al. Arthrodesis as an early alternative to nonoperative management of charcot arthropathy of the diabetic foot. J Bone Joint Surg Am 2000;82-A(7):939–50.

49. Mittlmeier T, Klaue K, Haar P, et al. Should one consider primary surgical reconstruction in Charcot arthropathy of the feet? Clin Orthop Relat Res 2010;468(4): 1002–11.

50. Kroin E, Chaharbakhshi EO, Schiff A, et al. Improvement in quality of life following operative correction of midtarsal charcot foot deformity. Foot Ankle Int 2018; 39(7):808–11.

51. Frykberg RG, Wittmayer B, Zgonis T. Surgical management of diabetic foot infections and osteomyelitis. Clin Podiatr Med Surg 2007;24(3):469–82, viii-ix.

52. Shaikh N, Vaughan P, Varty K, et al. Outcome of limited forefoot amputation with primary closure in patients with diabetes. Bone Joint J 2013;95-B(8):1083–7.

53. Raglan M, Dhar S, Scammell B. Is stimulan (synthetic calcium sulphate tablets impregnated with antibiotics) superior in the management of diabetic foot ulcers with osteomyelitis compared with standard treatment? Paper presented at: BOFAS annual meeting. Guildford, November 11-13, 2015.

54. Karr JC. Management in the wound-care center outpatient setting of a diabetic patient with forefoot osteomyelitis using Cerament Bone Void Filler impregnated with vancomycin: off-label use. J Am Podiatr Med Assoc 2011;101(3):259–64.

55. Jogia RM, Modha DE, Nisal K, et al. Use of highly purified synthetic calcium sulfate impregnated with antibiotics for the management of diabetic foot ulcers complicated by osteomyelitis. Diabetes Care 2015;38(5):e79–80.

56. Tiruveedhula M, Graham A, Dindyal S, et al. Midfoot Charcot—new staging system based on disease progression. The multidisciplinary orthopaedic and vascular reconstruction of the diabetic foot; 25/26/2019, 2019; London.

57. Brodsky JW, Rouse AM. Exostectomy for symptomatic bony prominences in diabetic charcot feet. Clin Orthop Relat Res 1993;(296):21–6.

58. Catanzariti AR, Mendicino R, Haverstock B. Ostectomy for diabetic neuroarthropathy involving the midfoot. J Foot Ankle Surg 2000;39(5):291–300.

59. Botezatu I, Laptoiu D. Minimally invasive surgery of diabetic foot–review of current techniques. J Med Life 2016;9(3):249.

60. Baravarian B, Van Gils CC. Arthrodesis of the Charcot foot and ankle. Clin Podiatr Med Surg 2004;21(2):271–89.

61. Zgonis T, Roukis TS, Lamm BM. Charcot foot and ankle reconstruction: current thinking and surgical approaches. Clin Podiatr Med Surg 2007;24(3):505–17, ix.

62. Jones CP. Beaming for Charcot foot reconstruction. Foot Ankle Int 2015;36(7): 853–9.

63. N. V, A. A, E. G, et al. Corrective mid foot fusion for Charcot neuroarthropathy–the Kings' experience. Orthop Proc 2016;98-B(SUPP_19):8.

64. Pinzur MS. Neutral ring fixation for high-risk nonplantigrade Charcot midfoot deformity. Foot Ankle Int 2007;28(9):961–6.

65. Wukich DK, Raspovic KM, Hobizal KB, et al. Radiographic analysis of diabetic midfoot charcot neuroarthropathy with and without midfoot ulceration. Foot Ankle Int 2014;35(11):1108–15.

66. Lamm BM, Stasko PA, Gesheff MG, et al. Normal foot and ankle radiographic angles, measurements, and reference points. J Foot Ankle Surg 2016;55(5):991–8.

67. Younger AS, Sawatzky B, Dryden P. Radiographic assessment of adult flatfoot. Foot Ankle Int 2005;26(10):820–5.

68. Ford SE, Cohen BE, Davis WH, et al. Clinical outcomes and complications of midfoot charcot reconstruction with intramedullary beaming. Foot Ankle Int 2019; 40(1):18–23.

69. Farber DC, Juliano PJ, Cavanagh PR, et al. Single stage correction with external fixation of the ulcerated foot in individuals with Charcot neuroarthropathy. Foot Ankle Int 2002;23(2):130–4.
70. Conway JD. Charcot salvage of the foot and ankle using external fixation. Foot Ankle Clin 2008;13(1):157–73, vii.
71. Egol KA, Kubiak EN, Fulkerson E, et al. Biomechanics of locked plates and screws. J Orthop Trauma 2004;18(8):488–93.
72. Marks RM, Parks BG, Schon LC. Midfoot fusion technique for neuroarthropathic feet: biomechanical analysis and rationale. Foot Ankle Int 1998;19(8):507–10.
73. Campbell JT, Schon LC, Parks BG, et al. Mechanical comparison of biplanar proximal closing wedge osteotomy with plantar plate fixation versus crescentic osteotomy with screw fixation for the correction of metatarsus primus varus. Foot Ankle Int 1998;19(5):293–9.
74. Schon LC, Easley ME, Weinfeld SB. Charcot neuroarthropathy of the foot and ankle. Clin Orthop Relat Res 1998;349:116–31.
75. Eschler A, Wussow A, Ulmar B, et al. Intramedullary medial column support with the Midfoot Fusion Bolt (MFB) is not sufficient for osseous healing of arthrodesis in neuroosteoarthropathic feet. Injury 2014;45(Suppl 1):S38–43.
76. Sammarco VJ, Sammarco GJ, Walker EW Jr, et al. Midtarsal arthrodesis in the treatment of Charcot midfoot arthropathy. J Bone Joint Surg Am 2009;91(1): 80–91.
77. Miller R. NEMISIS minimally invasive surgical correction for midfoot Charcot arthropathy. Foot & Ankle Orthopaedics 2018;3(3). 2473011418S2473000353.
78. Hastings MK, Mueller MJ, Sinacore DR, et al. Effects of a tendo-Achilles lengthening procedure on muscle function and gait characteristics in a patient with diabetes mellitus. J Orthop Sports Phys Ther 2000;30(2):85–90.
79. Hoke M. An operation for the correction of extremely relaxed flat feet. JBJS 1931; 13(4):773–83.
80. Schuberth JM, Babu-Spencer N. The impact of the first ray in the cavovarus foot. Clin Podiatr Med Surg 2009;26(3):385–93.

Correction of Severe Hallux Valgus with Metatarsal Adductus Applying the Concepts of Minimally Invasive Surgery

Alon Burg, MD[a,b,*], Ezequiel Palmanovich, MD[c]

KEYWORDS

- Hallux valgus • Metatarsus adductus • Minimally invasive surgery
- Proximal metatarsal osteotomy

KEY POINTS

- Hallux valgus associated with metatarsus adducts is a challenging deformity to correct.
- A normal or reduced intermetatarsal angle is the most critical part of the deformity, and impedes the displacement of the first metatarsal head.
- Current surgical techniques demonstrate low clinical and radiological outcomes when compared with a simple hallux valgus.
- Proximal lesser metatarsal osteotomies in a minimally invasive surgery allows correction the deformity.

INTRODUCTION

Hallux valgus (HV) is one of the most common pathologies of the forefoot, for which a multifactorial etiology has been proposed. Clinically, patients present with a painful medial bump, medial deviation of the first ray, and lateral deviation and protonation of the big toe.[1] Metatarsus adductus (MA) is defined as a transverse plane deformity where the metatarsals are deviated medially in relation to the midfoot.[2] It is a congenital deformity of uncertain etiology and a prevalence of 1 to 2 per 1000 births,[3] which is characterized by adduction of the metatarsals, supination of the subtalar, joint and plantar flexion of the first ray.[4] It is usually associated with lesser toe deformities, such as lateral deviation of the toes. MA is highly correlated with HV. MA was found in 30% of patients who underwent HV surgery,[5] and the risk for development of HV

[a] Department of Orthopedic Surgery, Foot and Ankle Service, Rabin Medical Center, Derech Ze'ev Jabotinsky Street, 39, Petah Tikva 4941492, Israel; [b] Tel Aviv University, Tel Aviv, Israel; [c] Orthopedic Department, Meir Medical Service, Sackler University, Tel Aviv University, 59 Tchernichovsky Street, Kfar-Saba 4428164, Israel
* Corresponding author.
E-mail address: dr.alonburg@gmail.com

Foot Ankle Clin N Am 25 (2020) 337–343
https://doi.org/10.1016/j.fcl.2020.02.001
1083-7515/20/© 2020 Elsevier Inc. All rights reserved.

is increased 3.5-fold when MA is present.[3] The presence of MA also complicates the surgical treatment of HV. The adduction of the second metatarsal bone reduces the space between the first and second rays, which prevents displacement of the first ray and correction of the deformity.[3,6–8] Thus, the presence of MA increases the recurrence of the deformity to 30%.[5]

DEFORMITY ASSESSMENT

HV is defined as an HV angle (ie, the angle between the long axis of first metatarsal and proximal phalanx) of greater than 15°. Many methods have been described to assess the magnitude of MA.[9] Some methods were developed to asses MA in pediatric population, whereas others have been used in assessing adult feet. In HV surgery, the principle is to assess the true intermetatarsal angle, as it would be if the second metatarsus was in its correct position. Measuring the angle between the longitudinal axis of the lesser tarsus and that of the second metatarsal using a modified Sgarlato's technique, that is, by using the fifth metatarsocuboid joint as a reference.[10,11] A normal value is an angle of 0° to 15°, mild MA is 16° to 19°, moderate MA is 20° to 25°, and severe MA is an angle of greater than 25°. Another popular method is to measure the Engel's angle, using a line bisecting the second cuneiform as a reference.[12] The Kilmartin angle is used to assess the true intermetatarsal angle by referencing the line parallel to the lateral border of the calcaneus, through the base of the second metatarsus.[13] (**Fig. 1**).

Correction of the Deformity

Although many surgical techniques have been described for HV correction, only a few methods are described for the treatment of HV in patients presenting with MA. Larholt and Kilmartin[7] reported a series of 27 patients who were treated with rotational scarf and akin osteotomy, without addressing the lesser metatarsals, and found their method to have satisfactory results, but with a high percentage (42%) of a HV angle

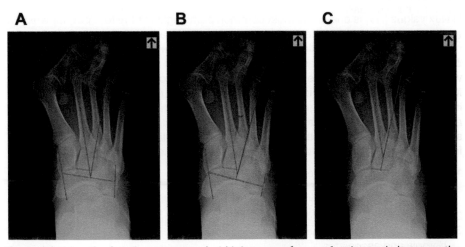

Fig. 1. (*A*) Using the fourth metatarsocuboid joint as a reference for the angle between the tarsal bones to the second metatarsus. (*B*) Sgarlato's technique, using the fifth metatarsocuboid joint as a reference for the angle between the tarsal bones to the second metatarsus. (*C*) Engel's angle, using a line bisecting the second cuniform as a reference for the angle between the tarsal bones to the second metatarsus.

of greater than 15° the end of follow-up. According to their study, the HV angle was reduced from 34.6° to 13.2°. Patient satisfaction was high, with 89% of patients being satisfied. Their study limitation, however, was a relatively high percentage of patients lost to follow-up. The authors acknowledged "the possibility that the adducted position of the metatarsals will create a residual valgus angle of the MTP joint." In a smaller series of 4 patients, an extensive treatment algorithm addressing the whole forefoot deformity was described, using osteotomies and rigid fixation of the lesser metatarsals. The approach yielded good clinical and radiographic outcomes; yet, it required a postoperative non-weight-bearing period of 6 weeks, followed by controlled weight bearing using a boot.[6] This surgical technique addresses the core issue of MA-associated HV. It gives an excellent correction of the entire deformity. However, this procedure can be very challenging. Although the authors did not report any cases of residual metatarsalgia, it has a potential for transfer metatarsalgia owing to the rigid fixation of the lesser metatarsals, which can cause sagittal imbalance. A case report by Martinelli and colleagues[14] described multiple distal oblique osteotomies of the first 3 metatarsals, with Z-lengthening of the long extensor tendons. Finally, another case report by Gordillo-Fernandez and colleagues[15] described a scarf osteotomy combined with distal lesser metatarsal osteotomies, and interphalangeal arthrodesis of the central toes with Z-lengthening of the capsule and long extensor tendons of the toes. These open surgeries techniques are very demanding, requiring a large exposure for the proximal osteotomy of the first ray and additional incisions for the toe shortening surgery that involve large scars, stiffness and other soft tissue damage, and a potential for increased risk of infections and nonunion or malunion.

In recent years, there has been a conceptual shift regarding bunion surgery. Instead of proximal osteotomies for larger deformities, it is becoming more common to perform distal osteotomies with large metatarsal head displacement.[16] Concurrently, minimally invasive surgery is growing in popularity, providing surgeons with new technique options that are based on these new concepts. The authors have developed a technique for treating HV associated with MA, by performing proximal metatarsal osteotomies in the second to fourth metatarsals, using the unique concepts of minimally invasive surgery.

SURGICAL PROCEDURE

The authors have devised a simple yet effective procedure to correct HV associated with MA. Our preliminary results were presented in the 2019 The Baltimore Alumnus Meeting (Burg A., Palmanovich E. Correction of HV deformity associated with MA using minimally invasive surgery concepts. Unpublished data. 2019 The Baltimore Alumnus Meeting, Breckenridge, Colorado). All procedures were performed under ankle block and with the use of fluoroscopy. HV associated with MA was treated as follows.

1. The lesser metatarsals were addressed first. A percutaneous lateral closing wedge osteotomy of the base of the second, third, and sometimes fourth metatarsal was performed. The medial cortex was usually preserved to be used as a hinge.
2. The lesser metatarsals were angled laterally to make room for the first ray (**Fig. 2**).
3. A minimally invasive chevron and akin procedure was performed, as described by Vernois and associates.[17–19] A percutaneous distal osteotomy was performed, followed by a lateral deviation of the metatarsal head and fixation with screws. An additional percutaneous akin procedure was done when necessary. The head was pushed as far laterally as needed to correct the true intermetatarsal angle, pushing the lesser metatarsals lateral.

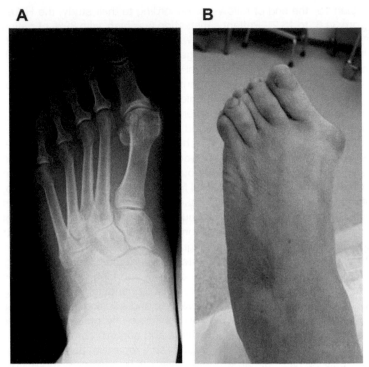

Fig. 2. (*A*) Preoperative radiograph of left foot of patient with HV associated with MA. (*B*) Clinical picture of same patient. Notice the severe HV with laterally deviated lesser toes.

4. A percutaneous varus closing wedge osteotomy of the second, third, and fourth proximal phalanges was performed. This addresses the laterally deviated toes (**Fig. 3**).
5. A second, distal metatarsal osteotomy was added in cases of severely prominent metatarsal head preoperatively or metatarsal phalangeal joint dislocation,
6. The medial stab wounds were sutured with rapid Vicryl sutures,
7. The foot was bandaged to maintain the position of the lesser toes.

POSTOPERATIVE MANAGEMENT

The operated feet were placed in a flat postoperative shoe and patients were advised to keep the foot elevated. The patients were permitted to bear weight as tolerated. Two weeks after the surgery, the bandages were changed and the wounds were inspected. Bandages were kept for 4 more weeks and then the patient converted to a normal shoe. The follow-up duration was at least 6 months (**Fig. 4**).

The authors reported functional outcome and satisfaction; complications and recurrence were also evaluated. After the consolidation, the realignment of the metatarsals was conserved. Complications included 2 patients who required a screw removal owing to prominence of the head under the skin, and 1 patient with a recurrent hammertoe (without recurrence of coronal deformity). There were no complaints of transfer metatarsalgia postoperatively.

The main concern when performing a rigidly fixed lateral closing wedge osteotomy of the lesser metatarsus is sagittal and length imbalance, producing metatarsalgia.

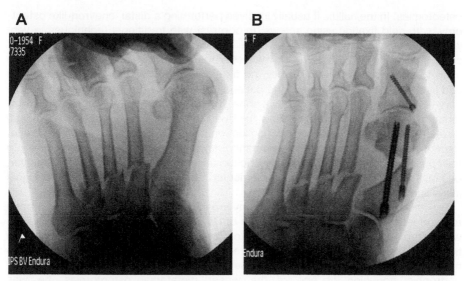

Fig. 3. (A) Intraoperative fluoroscopy demonstrating proximal metatarsal osteotomies to eliminate the MA and make room for the first metatarsal osteotomy. (B) Intraoperative fluoroscopy after performing the minimally invasive chevron and akin procedure for the first ray and the varus osteotomy of the proximal phalanges of the lesser toes.

Also, when using rigid fixation, one commits the patient to partial heel or non-weight-bearing for several weeks, until consolidation commences. By addressing these issues, minimally invasive surgery of the forefoot is becoming an extensively used approach.[20] It involves using a low-speed burr through stab wounds to create

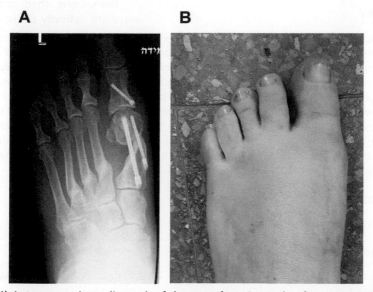

Fig. 4. (A) Anteroposterior radiograph of the same foot, 9 months after surgery. Notice all the osteotomies have healed and the metatarsus adductus angle is corrected along with the HV angle. (B) Clinical picture of same foot. notice correction of axis of all the toes.

osteotomies. In the hallux, it usually involves performing a distal, chevron-like osteotomy, with rigid fixation using screws. In contrast with traditional techniques, a very large bone displacement of up to 100% can be achieved, with good results and consolidation of the osteotomy. In the lesser toes, osteotomies and tenotomies are used to correct deformities. Usually, no fixation is used, apart from the bandages and sometimes internal sutures, and patients can bear weight immediately after surgery with a specialized postoperative shoe. In cases of metatarsalgia, a distal metatarsal osteotomy is indicated to allow the head to find the correct height, or sagittal position, during the process of consolidation, and full weight bearing is allowed. Because the osteotomy is done percutaneously, the metatarsals remain relatively in their position without fixation, so no restriction on weight bearing is needed. Moreover, because all of the correction is extra-articular, stiffness in the metatarsophalangeal joints is not encountered.

These concepts of metatarsal osteotomy are the novel minimally invasive approach for forefoot reconstruction and correction of HV in the presence of MA. In our series, we performed proximal metatarsal osteotomies before the bunion surgery, to realign the metatarsals. Once the metatarsals were displaced laterally, space for the displacement of the first metatarsal head was achieved. Although 1 patient presented with hypertrophic nonunion of one of the lesser metatarsal osteotomies, he was asymptomatic and did not require any treatment. The final follow-up showed that the realignment of the metatarsals was conserved. Our technique is very easy to perform for a surgeon with experience in minimally invasive surgery of the forefoot. Particularly, there is no need for fixation of the lesser metatarsals, and immediate weight bearing is permitted and encouraged. Because the metatarsal osteotomies are not fixed, the surgeon does not have to consider sagittal realignment because the metatarsal heads find their correct sagittal position with weight bearing. Breeching of the medial cortex seems to have no effect on this. These issues are addressed as the patient bears weight and healing commences.

SUMMARY

HV associated with MA is a surgical challenge with a high incidence of recurrence. Several methods have been proposed to deal with this difficult deformity. The authors presented proximal metatarsal osteotomies aimed at realigning the metatarsal in MA foot before correction of HV. Although the osteotomies were not fixed, the fusion rate was almost 100% and metatarsal alignment was conserved after fusion. This realignment created enough space for the bunion surgery, thereby improving the position of the foot.

We assert that this novel implementation of the minimally invasive concepts is an effective, safe, and reproducible technique for the treatment of HV associated with MA. We believe this technique addresses and successfully deals with the challenges of treating this difficult scenario.

DISCLOSURE

The authors have nothing to disclose.

REFERENCES

1. Fraissler L, Konrads C, Hoberg M, et al. Treatment of hallux valgus deformity. EFORT Open Rev 2016;1(8):295–302.
2. Dawoodi AI, Perera A. Reliability of metatarsus adductus angle and correlation with hallux valgus. Foot Ankle Surg 2012;18(3):180–6.

3. Loh B, Chen JY, Yew AKS, et al. Prevalence of metatarsus adductus in symptomatic hallux valgus and its influence on functional outcome. Foot Ankle Int 2015;36: 1316–21.

4. Harley BD, Fritzhand AJ, Little JM, et al. Abductory midfoot osteotomy procedure for metatarsus adductus. J Foot Ankle Surg 1995;34(2):153–62.

5. Aiyer AA, Shariff R, Ying L, et al. Prevalence of metatarsus adductus in patients undergoing hallux valgus surgery. Foot Ankle Int 2014;35(12):1292–7.

6. Sharma J, Aydogan U. Algorithm for severe hallux valgus associated with metatarsus adductus. Foot Ankle Int 2015;36:1499–503.

7. Larholt J, Kilmartin TE. Rotational scarf and akin osteotomy for correction of hallux valgus associated with metatarsus adductus. Foot Ankle Int 2010;31:220–8.

8. Coughlin MJ, Roger A. Mann Award. Juvenile hallux valgus: etiology and treatment. Foot Ankle Int 1995;16:682–97.

9. Marshall N, Ward E, Williams CM. The identification and appraisal of assessment tools used to evaluate metatarsus adductus: a systematic review of their measurement properties. J Foot Ankle Res 2018;11:25.

10. Dominguez G, Munuera PV. Metatarsus adductus angle in male and female feet: normal values with two measurement techniques. J Am Podiatr Med Assoc 2008; 98:364–9.

11. Sgarlato TE. Compendium of podiatric biomechanics. San Francisco (CA): California College of Podiatric Medicine; 1971.

12. Engel E, Erlick N, Krems I. A simplified metatarsus adductus angle. J Am Podiatry Assoc 1983;73:620–8.

13. Kilmartin T, Flintham C. Hallux valgus surgery: a simple method for evaluating the 1st 2nd Intermetatarsal angle in the presence of metatarsus adductus. J Foot Ankle Surg 2003;42:165–7.

14. Martinelli N, Marinozzi A, Cancilleri F, et al. Hallux valgus correction in a patient with metatarsus adductus with multiple distal oblique osteotomies. J Am Podiatr Med Assoc 2010;100:204–8.

15. Gordillo-Fernandez LM, Ortiz-Romero M, Macias JLSMS, et al. Surgical reconstruction of the forefoot with hallux valgus associated with metatarsus adductus. J Am Podiatr Med Assoc 2016;106:289–93.

16. Palmanovich E, Myerson MS. Correction of moderate and severe hallux valgus deformity with a distal metatarsal osteotomy using an intramedullary plate. Foot Ankle Clin 2014;19(2):191–201.

17. Vernois J, Redfern DJ. Percutaneous surgery for severe hallux valgus. Foot Ankle Clin 2016;21(3):479–93.

18. Kitaoka HB, Alexander IJ, Adelaar RS, et al. Clinical rating systems for the ankle-hindfoot, midfoot, hallux, and lesser toes. Foot Ankle Int 1994;15(7):349–53.

19. Ho B, Houck JR, Flemister AS, et al. Preoperative PROMIS scores predict postoperative success in foot and ankle patients. Foot Ankle Int 2016;37(9):911–8.

20. Cazeau C, Stiglitz Y. Minimally invasive and percutaneous surgery of the forefoot current techniques in 2018. Eur J Orthop Surg Traumatol 2018;28:819–37.

Moving?

Make sure your subscription moves with you!

To notify us of your new address, find your **Clinics Account Number** (located on your mailing label above your name), and contact customer service at:

Email: journalscustomerservice-usa@elsevier.com

800-654-2452 (subscribers in the U.S. & Canada)
314-447-8871 (subscribers outside of the U.S. & Canada)

Fax number: 314-447-8029

**Elsevier Health Sciences Division
Subscription Customer Service
3251 Riverport Lane
Maryland Heights, MO 63043**

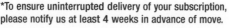